PENGUIN BOOKS

# Unnatural Causes

Dr Richard Shepherd was born in West London but grew up in Watford. At the local grammar school he was introduced to a medical textbook smuggled into the classroom by a friend, which opened his eyes to the world of crime and murder, setting him on a lifelong quest to understand death in its many forms. He trained as a doctor at St George's Hospital medical school at Hyde Park Corner, qualifying in 1977, and then completed his postgraduate training as a forensic pathologist in 1987. He immediately joined what was then the elite forensic department at Guy's Hospital.

He has been involved nationally and internationally in the forensic investigation of thousands of deaths from unnatural causes, from headline-making murders to mass natural disasters, and many sudden and unexplained deaths that his investigations showed were from natural causes or due to accidents. His skills and expertise still remain in demand around the world.

# Unnatural Causes

## DR RICHARD SHEPHERD

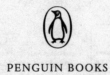

PENGUIN BOOKS

PENGUIN BOOKS

UK | USA | Canada | Ireland | Australia
India | New Zealand | South Africa

Penguin Books is part of the Penguin Random House group of companies
whose addresses can be found at global.penguinrandomhouse.com

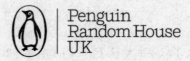

First published by Michael Joseph 2018
First published in Penguin Books 2019
007

Set in 12.5/14.75 pt Garamond MT Std
Typeset by Jouve (UK), Milton Keynes
Printed and bound in Great Britain by Clays Ltd, Elcograf S.p.A.

A CIP catalogue record for this book is available from the British Library

ISBN: 978-1-405-92353-8

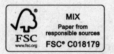

# Author's note

It was difficult for me to take the decision to change names and identifying details in this book because I've spent a working life striving for accuracy. However, I've also spent a working life trying to alleviate the suffering of the bereaved and it would help no one to recognize a relative in these pages and revisit their darkest days here. So only the names of those who are so famous they are impossible to disguise are given. In all other cases I have changed details to preserve confidentiality while maintaining relevant facts.

'Tis not enough, Taste, Judgement, Learning, join;
In all you speak, let Truth and Candour shine:
That not alone what to your Sense is due,
All may allow; but seek your Friendship too.
Be silent always when you doubt your Sense;
And speak, tho' sure, with seeming Diffidence:
Some positive, persisting Fops we know,
Who, if once wrong, will needs be always so;
But you, with Pleasure own your Errors past,
And make each Day a Critick on the last.
'Tis not enough your Counsel still be true;
Blunt Truths more Mischief than nice Falsehoods do;
Men must be taught as if you taught them not;
And Things unknown propos'd as Things forgot.
Without Good Breeding, Truth is disapprov'd;
That only makes Superior Sense belov'd.
Be Niggards of Advice on no Pretence;
For the worst Avarice is that of Sense:
With mean Complacence ne'er betray your Trust,
Nor be so Civil as to prove Unjust.
Fear not the Anger of the Wise to raise;
Those best can bear Reproof, who merit Praise.

Alexander Pope, *An Essay on Criticism*

# I

Clouds ahead. Some were snowy mountains looming over me. Others lay across the sky like long, sleeping giants. I moved the controls so gently that when the plane tilted down and to the left it seemed to respond not to command but by instinct. Then, ahead of me, the horizon straightened. It is a strange friend: always there, glimmering between sky and land, unapproachable, untouchable.

Beneath were the North Downs, their gentle curves bearing an odd similarity to the rise and fall of the human body. Now they were sliced cleanly through by the motorway. Cars chased each other along its deep cut. They gleamed like tiny fish. Then the M4 was gone and the earth was falling away towards water, a river knitted with a complexity of tributaries.

And here a town, its centre robust, red-hearted, radiating roads lined by paler, more modern buildings.

I swallowed.

The town was disintegrating.

I blinked.

An earthquake?

The town's colours waved. Its buildings were pebbles on a riverbed, viewed through the distorting lens of flowing water.

Extraordinary air currents?

No. Because the town waved in time with something inside me, something like nausea. But more ominous.

I blinked harder and my hand tightened on the plane's controls as if I could correct this feeling by correcting altitude or direction. But it came from deep inside me, forcing its way up through my body with a physical power that left me breathless.

I am a practical, sensible man. I looked for practical, sensible explanations. What had I eaten for breakfast? Toast? Harmless enough and offering no explanation for the sudden intensity of this sickness. And if it wasn't exactly nausea, then what? Its chief component was an inexplicable sense of unhappiness, and . . . yes, dread. A sense that something terrible was about to happen. Even . . . an urge to make it happen.

A ludicrous, irrational thought crossed my mind. What if I got out of the aeroplane?

I struggled with myself to remain seated, to keep breathing, to control the plane, to blink. To be normal again.

And then I glanced at the GPS. And read: Hungerford.

Red, older houses at the centre. Hungerford. On its peripheries, grey streets and playing fields. Hungerford.

And then it was gone, replaced by Savernake Forest, a vast green cushion of vegetation. Gradually the great forest brought me relief, as if I were a foot-traveller enjoying its leafy shade. If my heart rate was still raised the cause was retrospective horror. What had happened to me back there?

I am in my sixties. As a forensic pathologist, I have performed more than 20,000 post-mortems. But this recent experience was the first time in my entire career that I suspected my job, which has introduced me to the human body in death after illness, decomposition, crime, massacre, explosion, burial and pulverizing mass disasters, might have emotional repercussions.

Let's not call it a panic attack. But it shocked me into asking myself questions. Should I see a psychologist? Or even a psychiatrist? And, more worryingly, did I want to stop doing this work?

## 2

The Hungerford massacre, as it became known, was my first major case as a forensic pathologist and came absurdly soon after I began my career. I was young and keen and it had taken many years to qualify. Years of highly specialized training, far beyond routine anatomical and pathological study. I must admit that so much time spent staring at minute cellular differences on microscope slides nearly bored me into giving it up. On many occasions I had to reinspire myself by sneaking into the office of my forensic mentor, Dr Rufus Crompton. He let me read through his files and look at the booklets of photographs from his cases and sometimes I'd sit there, engrossed, long into the evening. And by the time I left I could remind myself why I was doing all this.

At last I qualified. I was rapidly installed at Guy's Hospital, in the Department of Forensic Medicine, under the wing of the man who was then the UK's best-known pathologist, Dr Iain West.

In those days, the late 1980s, pathologists were expected to join senior police officers as hard-drinking, tough-talking, alpha males. Those who carry out necessary work that repulses others often feel entitled to walk with a swagger in their step and Iain had that swagger. He was a charismatic man, an excellent pathologist and a bull in the witness box who was not scared to lock horns with counsel. He knew how to drink, charm women and hold a public bar spellbound with a good story. Although sometimes rather shy, I had almost convinced myself I was socially competent until I found myself playing the gawky younger brother to Iain. His light shone in pubs across London and I stood with an admiring audience in his shadow, seldom daring to risk adding a quip of my own. Or perhaps that was just because I couldn't think of a good one, anyway not until at least an hour later.

Iain was head of department and it was quite clear that he was top dog. The Hungerford massacre was a significant national disaster and a personal tragedy for the people of that town, especially those families directly affected. Under normal circumstances, Iain, as boss, would rush to such an event. But it was mid-August and he was on holiday so, when the call came, I took it.

I was driving home from work when my bleeper went off. It is difficult to imagine now that we lived in a world without mobiles but in 1987 there was nothing more than a single bleep to alert me to the fact that I should make a phone call as soon as I could. I switched on the radio, just in case the bleep was related to a headline. And found it was.

A gunman had been on the loose around a town in Berkshire so obscure that I had never visited and barely heard of it. He had been on a killing spree, starting in the Savernake Forest and working his way towards Hungerford town centre, and now he had retreated into a school building and the police had surrounded him. They were trying to persuade him to give himself up. Reporters believed that he may have killed as many as ten people, but since the town was under a sort of curfew there was no way of obtaining an accurate figure.

I arrived home, which in those days was a nice house in Surrey. A happy marriage, a nanny, two small children playing in the garden: it couldn't have contrasted more with the houses of murder scenes I visited. On that day, I knew my wife, Jen, probably wouldn't be there yet because she was busy studying.

I walked through the front door and straight to the phone, saying goodbye to the nanny as she left. I got the up-to-the-minute information and discussed with the police and coroner's office whether I needed to go to Hungerford this evening. They were adamant that I must. I promised to leave as soon as my wife returned.

Switching on the radio news, I listened to Hungerford updates while I made the children tea. Then I bathed them, read a story and tucked them into bed.

'Sleep well,' I said. I always did.

I was the caring parent focusing on his children. And simultaneously the forensic expert desperate to get in the car and see what was happening in the biggest case of his professional life so far. When Jen walked in, the forensic expert took over entirely. I kissed her goodbye and sprinted straight out.

The CID had instructed me to leave the M4 at Junction 14 and wait on the slip road for my police escort. A few moments later a police car slid alongside mine and two grim faces turned to me.

They offered no greetings.

'Dr Shepherd?'

I nodded.

'Follow us.'

Of course, I'd been listening to the radio all the way and I already knew that the massacre had ended with the death of the gunman. He was twenty-seven-year-old Michael Ryan, who, for no reason anyone could discern, had roved Hungerford armed with two semi-automatic rifles and a Beretta pistol. He was dead now, either because he had turned a gun on himself or a marksman had saved him the trouble. Reporters were excluded, the injured had been taken to hospital, residents were indoors and the town had been left to the police and the dead.

We passed through a roadblock and I followed the police car very slowly along eerily empty streets. The last long rays of the evening's summer sun were passing across this ghost town, bathing it in a benign, warm light. Anyone alive was inside their home but there was no sense of their presence at the windows. No car moved apart from our own. No dog barked. No cat prowled through flower beds. Birds were silent.

As we twisted and turned through the town's small suburbs we passed a red Renault askew at the side of the road. A woman's body was slumped over the wheel. Further on, as we turned into Southside, were the smouldering remains of Ryan's house on the left. The road was blocked. A police officer's body sat motionless in his squad car. The car was riddled with bullet holes. A blue Toyota had collided with it and inside was another dead driver.

An elderly man lying by his garden gate in a pool of blood. On the road an elderly woman, dead. Face down. I knew from news reports that this must be Ryan's mother. She lay outside her burning house. Further on, a man on a path, dog lead in hand. The juxtaposition on that almost-dark August evening between the quotidian streets and the extraordinary random acts of killing that had taken place there was, frankly, surreal. Nothing at all like this had happened in the UK before.

At the police station we halted. My door slammed and then the officer's door slammed and after that the heavy silence resumed to cover, no, smother, Hungerford. It was a few years before I was to hear another such silence, the silence that follows horror. Usually the scene of a homicide is accompanied by the bustle of the living – uniformed officers, detectives, crime scene investigators, people rustling paperwork, taking pictures, making phone calls, guarding the door. But the enormity of that day's events seemed to have frozen Hungerford in a state I can only compare to rigor mortis.

The police station was more of a police house: anyway, it was being refurbished, with lumps of plaster on the ground and wires hanging. I must have been greeted. I must have shaken hands. But it seems to me, looking back, that the formalities were carried out in total silence.

It was soon completely dark and I was in a police vehicle, heading for the school where Michael Ryan had barricaded and then shot himself.

We glided very slowly down the still street, the headlights picking up a crashed car, its driver clearly visible, motionless. Once again, I climbed out to look. The light from my torch slid over the feet, the torso, the head. Well, there was no doubt here about the cause of death. A gunshot wound to the face.

We stopped at the next car and then a couple more.

The gunshot wounds were in a different place each time. Some people had been shot once, some had been shot again and again and again.

Recovery vehicles were waiting unobtrusively to take away the crashed cars when the police had documented them and removed the bodies. I turned to the officer driving me. My voice hit the silence like breaking glass.

'There's no need for me to see any more of the bodies in situ. There's no doubt about how they died so I can deal with it all at post-mortem.'

'We need you to take a look at Ryan, though,' he said.

I nodded.

At the John O'Gaunt School there were many more police officers.

I was briefed downstairs.

'He told us he had a bomb. We haven't searched him yet because we were worried that it would detonate if we moved him. But we need you to have a look at him now and certify death. Just in case he blows up when we do look. All right?'

'Right.'

'I suggest you don't move him, sir.'

'Right.'

'Do you want a flak jacket?'

I declined. It was designed to stop bullets and so would have been of little use at such close range to a bomb. And, anyway, I had no intention at all of moving Ryan.

We went upstairs. That rubbery smell of school. And when they opened the classroom door, there were desks. Some of the desks were scattered but most still stood in neat rows. Pinned around the walls were pictures and scientific diagrams. All perfectly normal. Apart from a body, propped up in a sitting position at the front of the class near the blackboard.

The killer was dressed in a green jacket. He would have looked like a man off hunting for the day if there hadn't been a gunshot wound to his head. His right hand lay in his lap. It held a Beretta pistol.

As I set off towards him, I was aware that all the policemen were quietly leaving. I heard the door close behind me. From beyond it there came a radio message: 'Going in.'

I was on my own in a classroom with the UK's biggest mass murderer. And perhaps a bomb. I had been attracted to my profession by the books of that lion of forensic pathology, Professor Keith Simpson. But I couldn't remember him mentioning this as a possibility in any of them.

I was acutely aware of everything around me. The quiet sounds beyond the door. The arc lights outside throwing overlapping, dark shadows on the ceiling. The small beam of my own torch. That classroom smell of chalk and sweat, mixed strangely with the smell of blood. I crossed the room, focusing on the body in the corner. On arrival, I knelt down to look at him. The gun, which had already killed so many people that day, was pointing straight at me.

Michael Ryan had shot himself in the right temple. The bullet had passed through his head and out of the other temple. I saw it later as I left the room, embedded in a noticeboard across the classroom.

I debriefed the officers. There were no hidden wires. The cause of death was the gunshot wound to the right side of the head, which was typical of suicide.

Then, relieved to be leaving that sad grave of a place,

I gathered speed on the motorway. But it seemed that Hungerford's silence had infiltrated the car and was riding alongside me, a massive and unwanted passenger. Suddenly I was overwhelmed by all I had seen that day. The enormity of it. The horror. I pulled over to the hard shoulder and sat in the dark car while the lights of other vehicles swept by, unseeing, unknowing.

I only became aware of the police car which had pulled up behind me when there was a tap at the window.

'Excuse me, sir. Are you all right?'

I explained who I was and where I'd been. The officer nodded, scrutinizing me, assessing me, wondering whether to believe me.

'I just need a minute,' I said, 'before I continue.'

Police officers know about transitions between work and home. He nodded again and returned to his own car. No doubt to check my story. A few quiet minutes later and I knew I had left Hungerford behind and home was ahead. I indicated, waved goodbye and rejoined the great river of motorway traffic. The police car pulled out behind me, following me protectively for a short distance before dropping back then turning off. I continued my journey alone.

At home, the children were in bed and Jen was downstairs, watching TV.

'I know where you've been,' she said. 'Was it awful?'

Yes. But I only allowed myself to shrug. I turned my back to her so that she could not see my face. I felt I had to extinguish the television news with its reporters discussing Hungerford excitedly and so urgently. The Hungerford dead had no excitement or urgency any more. Here were men and women simply slaughtered as they went about life's business, business they thought important and pressing until it was brought to an abrupt halt. There was nothing important for them now. There was nothing pressing.

Late into the night I was busy making phone calls to sort out how I would conduct multiple post-mortems the next day. I hoped to help the police reconstruct every death and thus, with witness help, all Ryan's moves. Reconstruction is important. It matters a lot to anyone involved, and it matters to the wider world. As humans, we have a need to know. About specific deaths. About death in general.

The following morning I performed some routine post-mortems: drunks, drug addicts and heart attacks, all at Westminster mortuary. While my colleagues asked me for details of Hungerford, the police there were moving the last bodies to the mortuary at the Royal Berkshire Hospital in Reading. When I arrived at about 2 p.m. I was greeted by the staff and then got to know them in our business's time-honoured fashion, over a cup of tea. A brew was and is regarded as a mortuary essential, both a right and a duty before performing a post-mortem.

And then the door swung open and Pam Derby bustled in. The room was filled with movement. Pam was our diminutive but crucially important secretary.

'Right!' she said.

Always a commanding presence, she was now looking at her most formidably efficient. Two unhappy mortuary assistants struggled behind her with the computer.

'Where can I plug in?'

This wasn't a question, it was a demand. Office computers

were in their infancy in 1987 and they were very large infants. In fact, ours must have hatched from a dinosaur egg as Pam had to bring it down from Guy's in a van.

She saw that I was in my green apron and white wellies, just starting to get the external examinations and X-rays organized. I was ready to go.

'No, no, no, you can't start until the computer's warmed up and it takes at least ten minutes or you'll get too far ahead of me. Make me a cup of tea,' she instructed. Iain West was clearly deluding himself that he ran the department.

While the computer and the kettle whirred, Pam sat down at the keyboard.

'Not much point in all this nonsense; they've been shot, anyone can see that,' she said briskly. Pam was familiar with the emotional, unplanned chaos of real homicides. That's why she and the other staff, for relaxation, often read neatly plotted whodunits, where the murderer leaves clear clues and at the end the pieces of the jigsaw click into place. It's all so different from the many versions of the truth, the conflicting facts and interpretations of them which are the messy face of real investigations.

She was right, there were no mysteries ahead today. But each case was a sibling, a parent, a child, a lover. Each was special to family and friends and each presented a unique puzzle for me to solve. The six tables stretched to the end of the room with a body on alternate surfaces: the empty tables in between were to be used for bagging and documenting the hundreds of exhibits we were going to take.

The first body was Michael Ryan. Probably most bereaved relatives did not wish him to share a mortuary with his victims, let alone a post-mortem room. In fact, everyone just wanted him to go. The press was still hinting with smug glee that he had been 'taken out' by the SAS – despite the police press release which confirmed, after my visit the night before, that he had committed suicide. Now we also needed to say that the post-mortem confirmed his suicide.

A post-mortem, also called an autopsy, is carried out in two situations. It may be performed after a natural death, usually in hospital, despite the cause of death being known, to confirm the patient's medical diagnosis and, possibly, examine the effects of treatment. The deceased's immediate family will be asked to agree to a post-mortem and will have an absolute right to decline. Fortunately, many agree. Their decision can help other patients by giving medical staff a superb opportunity to learn and improve. Agreeing to such a request for a post-mortem is, I think, a very generous act.

The second situation occurs when the cause of death is unknown or where there is a possibility it is unnatural. In this case, the death is referred to the coroner. All suspicious, unnatural, criminal or unexplained deaths have not just a post-mortem but a forensic post-mortem. This is a complete and extremely detailed investigation of the outside and the inside of the body. Afterwards these details are recorded by the pathologist in the post-mortem report.

The report must confirm the formal identification of the deceased and this alone is often a very long and complex process, and one which occasionally can never be completed. The report also explains why the post-mortem was requested by the police or the coroner. It lists those present while it was carried out. It gives details of any subsequent laboratory tests.

The bulk of the report is a description of exactly what the pathologist has found. We usually offer some interpretation of these findings and at the end we give a cause of death. If we don't know why the person died we say so – although usually after discussing the possibilities.

Despite all our years of training on the macro- and microscopic appearances of the organs in thousands of diseases, just looking carefully at the body before us is often the most vital part of the post-mortem. During this detailed external examination, we measure and record the size, location and shape of every scratch and bruise as well as any bullet holes and stab wounds. This may seem simple compared with our medical analysis of the body's interior but it has often proved the most important part of reconstructing a homicide. It is all too easy to regard external examination as a mere formality, and therefore to rush it. Then, long after a body has been cremated, we might regret those skimpy notes.

Michael Ryan was a mass murderer. He killed sixteen people and there were almost as many wounded. My career so far had focused on the victims of accidents, crime or just bad luck. I seldom saw perpetrators, and had certainly never seen someone who had caused so much death and injury. Could I, should I, treat Ryan with the same respect I showed his victims?

I knew I had to. Feelings have no place in the post-mortem room. I suspect that one of the greatest skills I have learned is not to feel a moral repulsion which others might think is not only justified but required. So whatever

I felt about this young man and his actions, I excluded that from my mind and my heart. I knew that his examination required as much, or maybe even more, care and attention than others. Only after a thorough and conclusive physical investigation could I furnish the coroner with the information he needed to confidently give the correct verdict at the inquest. I knew that proof was crucial for this verdict, to quell any future challenges or the inevitable conspiracy theories.

It was hard to imagine that the slender young man who lay naked on the post-mortem table had just finished a killing spree. Everyone in the room – police officers, mortuary staff, even Pam – stared at him with incomprehension. He looked as vulnerable as any victim of crime, as any of his own victims.

Then I got on with my job: fully to examine him, particularly the entry and exit wounds in his head. Next to open his body up for internal examination, taking samples for toxicology. And finally to trace the bullet's trajectory through his brain.

As I started work, the place was plunged into absolute and total silence. No calling. No rattling. No banging. No kettles or cups of tea. Just silence. Even the temperature seemed to drop significantly. As soon as I had finished, he was wheeled away. No one wanted to be near him, this strange young man who had lived quietly with his mother harbouring an obsession with firearms and thinking God knows what thoughts.

Now I started on Ryan's victims, and I could see it would be a long, hard, stressful day. Fridges clanged open and shut as we completed one post-mortem and started another. Apart from this, and my voice dictating to Pam, the room remained silent. I was helped by a trainee pathologist, Jeanette MacFarlane. Pam typed at my dictation and a rolling rota of photographers and police officers followed me from table to table, the most senior taking notes, others taking my exhibits.

Behind me the mortuary staff worked, cleaning bodies then sewing them up and preparing them for their families to see.

The deaths were straightforward, all from gunshot wounds. Not one victim had seen Ryan bristling with weapons and simply dropped dead from a heart attack. But it was my job to look for any natural disease that might have caused or hastened death. Once again, I had to carefully document each wound, describe it, analyse it, follow the trajectory of the bullet or bullets. I walked around each body, directing the photographer, measuring wounds, noting abnormalities, chanting my liturgy to Pam. Gradually a picture of Ryan's day of madness emerged.

Generally, victims who were killed with only one shot had been killed from a distance. If he got close to a victim, Michael Ryan apparently had the urge to fire more often.

When his mother, a dinner lady, heard from a friend what was going on, she came home to remonstrate with him. The friend drove her to Southside and she walked up the road towards their home, past injured and dead people, approaching her son fearlessly.

She said, 'Stop it, Michael!'

He faced her and shot her once in the leg with the

semi-automatic rifle. This brought her face-down on the ground. In my opinion, it was his intention only to maim her with that shot. He then walked up to her, stood over her and shot her twice in the back to kill her.

These last two shots showed the typical soot and burning around the wound when a weapon has been fired from close range, maybe from within six inches. Perhaps he simply could not look at her face as he murdered her. Until she arrived he had remained in the small area around his house and I personally formed the theory that her death released him to rampage much more widely through the town. I thought this had set him free to revel in the experience of an extraordinary and unaccustomed power, the power his weapons gave him over the unarmed.

Over the next few days I continued with my strange work, slowly moving from body to body. Death for these victims was an unexpected, violent end to peaceful and perhaps otherwise uneventful lives. Everyone in the mortuary was greatly moved by this, but we could not allow ourselves to give in to our sense of horror, or even to feel upset. Shock has no place in the work of a pathologist. We must seek the truth with clinical detachment. In order to serve society we sometimes have to suspend some aspects of our own humanity. I believe that same suspended humanity powerfully reasserted itself as I flew over Hungerford almost thirty years later.

In fact, it has taken me all this time to admit that I was very deeply affected by the massacre. I did not then acknowledge to myself shock or sadness, not in any way. My colleagues, alpha males or aspiring to be, were my role models, and they would never have shown or expressed such a thing, nor allowed themselves to think it. No, in order to do this work, I had to remember the professional integrity of the forensic pathologist Professor Keith Simpson that had inspired me in my teens to pursue my training. Was shock or horror something he ever wrote about? No it was not.

When Iain came back from holiday he did not ask me about Hungerford, he did not offer me advice or refer to the events there in any way at all. It is certain that he was livid with me for taking on such a huge case in his absence, although it was my job to cover his holiday period. Could I have located him to recall him from holiday? Perhaps, and, for this, he would certainly have come. We both knew that such a huge case should have been his: he had dealt with many IRA bombings and bullets; indeed, ballistics was his speciality.

The face of his fury was *froideur*, but gradually reports leaked out from colleagues that Iain believed one of the stupidest parts of Ryan's rampage was to do it while he, Iain, was on holiday. And among ourselves we added that, as if that wasn't stupid enough, Iain privately thought Ryan was an idiot to shoot himself, depriving the renowned Dr West of a spectacular court appearance.

For a long time, Hungerford lay between us, but there was no doubt my position at Guy's, and probably throughout the UK, shifted as a result of my work there. I was no longer the gawking, younger brother and doting follower of Iain. I was a noted forensic pathologist in my own right.

# 3

My strange, emotional flashback to the events of 1987 in Hungerford was all too easy to ignore once I had made the radio calls, turned the plane onto final approach and landed safely. It's a Cessna 172 that I share with a syndicate of twenty or so other people in Liverpool. It is my pleasure (and my madness, because door-to-door the train is nearly always quicker), to fly to meetings and postmortems in other parts of the UK and Ireland as often as I can.

I bounced along the landing strip at the grassy little airfield in broad sunshine, found my stand and shut down the engine. I left the Cessna and saw my colleague waiting for me. I felt fine. As we drove off I began to wonder if I had imagined that something had happened up there. Perhaps I had been short of oxygen in the cockpit? Well hardly, at 3,000 feet. Anyway, I was now sure my reaction could not have been as violent as I remembered. Not a panic attack at all, really.

As I flew back later, the more variable weather conditions demanded my undivided concentration and I hardly thought about Hungerford. Except to avoid it. It did occur to me then, for the first time, that the pilot's preoccupation with staying alive, which so powerfully suppresses all other thoughts, feelings and fears, may be one of the reasons I fly.

Home at last, the clouds cleared to reveal a soft summer's evening. I made myself a whisky and soda and sat outside on the patio to enjoy the last rays of the setting sun.

But suddenly, unexpectedly, the pearly summer dusk, and that hushed stillness which accompanied it, reminded me of . . . Hungerford. Again. My heart beat faster. I felt strangely lightheaded – and I hadn't taken one sip of my drink. Once more I was moving slowly through a small town's streets as bodies lay unmoving in pools of blood by lawnmowers, in cars, across the pavement. A sense of dread began to grip my chest and squeeze it hard.

I breathed deeply. To calm down. I reminded myself that I now knew what was happening. I had established my own mind was playing tricks. Obviously. So, with great effort, I must be able to control it. Obviously.

More breathing. Close my eyes. I had to crush this, crush it like ice inside curled fingers.

Gradually my body relaxed. My clenched fist loosened. My breathing deepened. I raised the glass unsteadily to my lips. Yes. Everything was back under control.

By the time I had drained the glass, I could safely answer the two questions I had asked myself in the plane that morning. No, of course I didn't need to see a psychologist, and certainly not a psychiatrist: the very idea seemed absurd. And there was no good reason for me to stop practising as a forensic pathologist either. Whatever was happening to me today would soon pass and all would be well. For sure.

A few months later, in the autumn of 2015, co-ordinated terrorist attacks on Paris bars, restaurants, a sports stadium and a music venue claimed 130 lives and injured hundreds of others. I was out on a call when I heard the radio news. Behind the reporter were the wails of sirens which accompany every emergency and the gabble of shocked voices. Horror's soundscape. I had to stop the car.

Sitting in a lay-by near my house, I closed my eyes. But they could still see, and my ears could hear. Ambulance blue lights. Police barriers. Rows of post-mortem tables under the bright mortuary glare, and on them human body parts. Shouting. Police radios. The cries of the wounded. Before me, bodies. In my nostrils, the smell of death. A foot, a hand, a child. A young woman who had been dancing in a nightclub, her intestines unwinding. Men in suits and ties but without legs. Office workers, tea ladies, students, pensioners. Destroyed, every one of them.

I don't know which of the disasters I have seen I was looking at now: the Bali bombs, the 7/7 London bombing, the Clapham rail disaster, the sinking of the *Marchioness*, 9/11 in New York, the Whitehaven massacre . . . or maybe it was all of them.

I waited at the roadside for the tidal wave that was engulfing me to subside. When it was over, I was left with a sense of misery and dread. The smell of human decay seemed to linger in the car for some minutes. I took deep breaths. It passed.

I drove off, shocked but under control.

Maybe I did need to discuss this with a professional after all. A priest, perhaps? Some person, anyway, whose job it is to receive our weaknesses and offer us strength.

Involuntarily I shook my head. Of course not. The events in Paris were terrible but I had not been called to help and they were nothing to do with me. I had a thorough understanding of death and no fear of it. The news from Paris had unexpectedly opened up a seam of memories, but the crevasse had closed again now. Aware of the long night of work that lay ahead of them, I just felt sorry for my French colleagues.

So I continued my journey. Off to the mortuary and business as usual. Surely I would be just fine.

# 4

From an early age I have had a relationship with death that is both intimate and distant. I come from a comfortable home near London. My father was a local authority accountant who had moved with my mother from the north of England to seek his fortune in the south. There was no fortune but we were well enough off: people who like categories would have called us lower middle-class. My sister is ten years older than me and my brother five. I was the loved baby of the family and we were unusual in only one respect. Our mother had a heart complaint that meant she was gradually fading away.

She had contracted rheumatic fever as a child and one of the complications of that childhood infection was that her mitral heart valve was progressively damaged. I know that now. Then, all I knew was that she was frequently breathless even after only a little exercise and, unlike other people's mothers, often had to sit down.

My big sister, Helen, assured me that my mother had once been a vibrant, laughing woman who mercilessly dragged my reluctant and rather dour father onto the dance floor at every opportunity. Who had set off as a young woman with him on a bicycle-built-for-two on a tour of Europe just when war was about to break out. Who was always the life and soul of the party.

I liked to sit in the living room listening to my sister's

stories about our mother. Walls, in those days, were rather bare, but carpets overcompensated for this in swirliness. In the corner was a tiny black-and-white television, one in which the white dot at the centre of the screen persisted when you switched off the picture, enduring mesmerizingly for several minutes in the dark. There was a radiogram (a huge combination of record player and wireless), its front covered in gauze, from which issued mainly light classical music of the type considered improving by the aspiring middle classes.

The electric fire glowed warmly, although probably with more light than heat. And the armchairs may have been worn but they were strategically covered by antimacassars. Yes, it was cheering to listen on the loud living-room carpet to tales of that lively woman. But she seemed to have nothing in common with the mother who often languished in bed. Upstairs. Or in hospital.

Her hospitalizations were long and frequent, at least that is how it seemed to me as a boy. I was often packed off to seaside holidays with my grandma in Lytham St Annes, or to my aunt in Stockport, and didn't discover until long afterwards that this wasn't so much for me to have fun on the beach or to see my cousin but to allow my mother time for surgery and convalescence.

At home with me, she certainly tried hard to be normal. She got up each morning and packed me lovingly off to school (even very young children walked to school alone in those days). It was only when, one day, I forgot my violin and returned unexpectedly to find her back in bed, that I realized she collapsed between the sheets each morning as soon as I left. She was as shocked to witness my discovery as I was to make it. I fear I was so taken aback that I even chided the poor woman. I wanted her to get better and be that mother everyone said she once had been. But even I could see that she was disappearing before my very eyes.

One day in December I came home from school and found her gone. She was in a hospital I now know to be the Royal Brompton. More tests and more bed rest. She was forty-seven.

I was taken to see her on Christmas Day. My memory of that visit has almost broken beneath the weight of subsequent memories of the many hospitals of my working life. I can dig down through the years, sifting geological strata, until I reach Christmas 1961, but what I find there breaks into fragments when I try to stare at it. It can only be captured in swift, sideways glances.

I was aware that nine-year-olds were generally not welcome on the wards. I was told to be on my best behaviour. Full of this knowledge, I was led down high, echoing corridors. Busy nurses in smart, starched uniforms scurried past us. On each side were vast rooms. A smell of disinfectant. Through faraway windows, the yellowing light of a dull London day. Turning suddenly behind my father into a large ward. Floorboards. A long line of beds, all white, all ready for the next patient. In my memory, all of them empty. Except for one. In it was my mother and, looking back, it seems to me she was the only patient on the ward for Christmas.

I wish I could remember how my mother greeted me, how she looked at me. I expect she hugged me and held my hand. I think she did. I expect I climbed on the bed and showed her the toys I'd received. Maybe I opened some presents with her. I think I did. I hope I did.

A few weeks later, on a cold January morning, I got up early as usual and left the room I shared with my brother, Robert, to cross into my parents' room and slide into bed with my father. I did that every morning. But today, something was wrong. The bed was cold. The sheets were still tidy. It had not been slept in.

I crept to the top of the stairs. Lights. Lights on in the house early in the morning. And voices. They weren't speaking normally, as if it were daytime. They were night-time hushed voices, their register strange, singing notes of alarm I didn't recognize. I stole back to bed and lay there. Waiting. Worrying. Something had happened and sooner or later someone would explain it to me.

Eventually, our father came in.

Horrifically, shockingly, he was crying. We stared at him, Robert blinking because he had just woken up.

Our father said, 'Your mother was a wonderful woman.'

At nine, that was too subtle for me. Robert had to explain the significance of the past tense, that our mother was in the past tense now. Because she was dead.

Eventually, I learned that my father and sister had gone to visit her as usual at the Royal Brompton the previous evening. She still wasn't well, but didn't seem any worse. They wished her goodnight as usual and were just leaving when the nurse took them aside and said, 'You do realize how ill the patient is? I'm afraid Mrs Shepherd probably won't last the night.'

This was shocking news because the possibility of her death had simply not occurred to anyone. If it had occurred to my father, or had been suggested to him by medical staff, he had convinced himself it wouldn't happen. She was in hospital to get better. Family visited her. That's how things were. No one anticipated an end to it.

In fact, she was a terminal cardiac case. She had heart failure and had now developed bronco-pneumonia, a disease which is often called Old Folks' Friend because it releases the weak from their suffering. She was certainly unable to withstand pneumonia, even though there were now antibiotics to treat that infection. If only penicillin had been discovered in time to prevent rheumatic fever from damaging her heart as a child.

Years later, when I was a medical student, my father solemnly produced her post-mortem report from some special drawer and asked me to explain it. I told him how her body's response to childhood rheumatic fever had made chemicals in the blood that killed the bacteria. But those chemicals had attacked not just the infection but also the body's own tissues – in this case, quite typically, the mitral valve of her heart. This valve, which controls the flow of blood through the left side of the heart, had become so scarred that it was stiff and jammed partly shut. Every time my mother went into hospital for open-heart surgery, the surgeons literally poked their fingers through the valve to free the valve cusps. Result: they flapped more normally again and blood flow between the left atrium and the left ventricle was restored. Or anyway, improved. For a while.

This was why she had so often disappeared to the hospital prostrate and returned reinvigorated. But each time the improvement was smaller.

This was pioneering open-heart surgery for its era, at the forefront of medical science, but it was no way to win a battle against a recalcitrant heart valve which the patient's own body was determined to destroy. Indeed, by the time I got to medical school ten years later, such treatment had already been superseded. Now she could have been fitted with a new, synthetic heart valve and survived, leading an active life for many more years.

I knew none of this at the time of my mother's death. I didn't know what I was supposed to feel, either. Everyone looked at me with tears in their eyes expecting something. But what? I went next door to my friend John's house. It was a Saturday and the whole family was there. His mother was warm and tearful and John and I sat watching television cartoons together. Even when they were funny, I thought I shouldn't laugh.

It all happened again soon afterwards when I came home from school and found the house full of relatives and flowers. I worked out later that the funeral had taken place; it had not crossed anyone's mind that I should go. When I walked in they looked at me tragically. What were they expecting me to do, to say? I felt nothing. Perhaps deep down I simply did not grasp the concept of death. My mother had so often disappeared before and had always come back. Possibly, despite appearances, I trusted her to return again.

When I look back on the early years of my life, on my mother, I remember little and feel nothing of her. Was this because of her frequent absences in hospital and strange lack of presence even when at home? How is it that I remember so much from that time about my grandmothers, my brother, sister, father, aunt . . . but there is a void where she should be? And I suppose there always will be.

After her death, the most surprising thing happened. My father changed. I think he analysed what we had lost and tried to supply it by becoming both mother and father. He stopped being dour and withdrawn and instead turned into an immensely loving man. My big sister helped a lot, although she was nineteen when my mother died and had already left home for teacher-training college. My father thought she might come back to look after the lads but, wisely, she did not – although she remained the most loving and supportive of elder sisters, even after her own marriage a few years later.

My father managed the house, shopping, cooking and working full-time in an era when there were few single fathers and consumerism was so undeveloped that shops were invariably closed when working people could visit them. He firmly believed it was possible to do anything you set your mind to. So, he rewired the house and painted the kitchen and serviced the car and learned to cook (with, admittedly, variable results). In addition, he somehow arranged his life to accommodate our needs and this involved his discovery of a new ability to give and receive great affection. I look back on all this and feel huge admiration for him.

There is a small black-and-white picture of my father with a large, leggy child, who must be me, enveloped in his lap. Both of us are asleep. This picture is most unusual for its time. Post-war men, on the whole, had been brought up by Victorian fathers and simply did not know how to show their sons such a degree of love and kindness.

He ensured I had a good childhood. I enjoyed school, passed my eleven-plus, loved swimming, went to the local youth club, sang in a choir and had a lot of friends. One of these friends was the son of a GP. When we were about thirteen, to spook us all, he 'borrowed' one of his father's medical books from the shelves at home and brought it to school. It was *Simpson's Forensic Medicine* (Third Edition) by Professor Keith Simpson, a small, tatty, red book which promised nothing on the outside. But inside, it was full of pictures of dead people. In fact, mostly murdered people. They were strangled, electrocuted, hanged, knifed, shot, asphyxiated . . . no hideous fate could escape Professor Simpson. He had seen everything. There was a photo of the fern-like pattern on the skin that a lightning strike can leave, a picture of the inside of the skull of a boy who had been hit on the head with a brick and an astonishing gallery of bullet entry and exit wounds as well as photos of bodies in various stages of decomposition.

I was, of course, by now all too familiar with the concept of death. I had personally experienced many of its repercussions. But I knew nothing about death's physical presentation. My mother had died in hospital far away and certainly no one had thought it appropriate for me to see her body. Even the most amateur psychologist must deduce that my need to explore death's presentation was the reason for my extraordinary interest in that copy of *Simpson's Forensic Medicine*. More than an interest, it was a fascination. It went further than prurience and much further than the other boys' eagerness to be horrified.

I borrowed the book and studied it for hours. I read and then reread the text and stared at the accompanying pictures. They were certainly graphic, especially since in those days no attempt was made to spare relatives, so victims' faces were not obscured.

Perhaps I wanted to view that horrifying thing, the worst that could happen, that thing called death, through the detached, clinical, analytical eyes of the great Simpson. Perhaps Simpson helped me to manage the unmanageable. Or perhaps I was simply excited by this mixture of medical knowledge and detective work.

I'd considered studying medicine. Pathology was interesting but forensic pathology was medicine and then some. I understood that, unlike other pathologists, the forensic pathologist does have patients. Unlike other doctors, though, all his patients are dead. And there certainly could be no comparison with the life of a GP, confronting a line of sniffing people every morning.

I learned that the forensic pathologist was called to any suspicious death at any time of the day or night, and that might mean to the actual scene of an actual murder. His job (it was always a he in those days) was to carry out a thorough medical analysis of the body to help police solve the crime. There could be a man lying dead of gunshot wounds and the pathologist would not only examine the scene and the wounds but also, said Simpson, at once demand to see any firearms found in the vicinity.

He must then ask himself four questions:

1. Could the wound have been inflicted with that weapon?

2. At what range was it fired?
3. From what direction?
4. Could the wound have been *self*-inflicted?

And for Professor Keith Simpson, that was all in a day's work. Thirsty to know more, I read as much as I could about him and fell in love with the way he rushed to crime scenes, often in those days by steam train, and then used his medical skills to help detectives reconstruct homicides, solve the unsolvable, exonerate the innocent, argue the case in court and bring to justice the perpetrator.

My future became clear to me after that. My lofty ambition was to become the next Professor Keith Simpson.

# 5

I was in an immense, clinical, white-tiled basement in Bloomsbury. Overhead, lights glared. Before me, under a sheet, its shape eerily discernible, lay the first dead body I would ever see.

All the medical students at University College London took Anatomy. There were about seventy freshers, and we knew what Anatomy meant. Dissection. I'd dissected a dogfish at school. Also a rat. Now we were going to dissect a human body.

When I walked down the stairs and smelled the formalin I recognized it at once from the school biology labs. We progressed through the room, passing perhaps forty porcelain tables where dissections were still in progress for the students from the years ahead of us. We threaded our way carefully, knowing that there were bodies under those sheets. Then, when I brushed past one, the sheet fell away at the corner to reveal a huge, hairy gorilla foot. Ha ha, just part of the Comparative Anatomy course. I laughed nervously. We all laughed nervously. Everyone was nervous.

For a lot of people, what we were about to do was scary or disgusting. My own anxiety was different. I was still determined to become a forensic pathologist like Professor Keith Simpson but I had actually only seen dead humans in photos. So how would I react to my first dead body? I knew that if I vomited, fainted, blanched or even faltered (and there were people in the room on the verge of doing all that), then the career I'd set my heart on would be over before it had begun.

Four to a table, wearing our new, crisp, white coats, we gathered around the bodies. These bodies would stay with us throughout our Anatomy course for eighteen months until we knew more about them physically than they could ever have known themselves – but less about them personally than any stranger who had shared a bus ride and seen their face in motion or heard their voice.

While we waited for the tutor, we all tried, in our different ways, to displace our emotions. But the unmistakable curves of those human forms, lifeless beneath the sheets, changed the dynamic in our group. There was a lot of bravado. Some made jokes, others felt obliged to laugh heartily. And eyes met, people held each other's gazes. A few invitations to date were blurted out. The room throbbed with intense personal relationships under this new and unaccustomed pressure.

Then the tutor started to speak and we stood to attention by our bodies. His words were received in deep, deep silence. The harsh light bounced off the tiles, off our lab coats, off the shiny scalpels and off our now tense, drained faces.

The sheets were removed and there they were. The dead. Grey, still, silent, unseeing. Some people fixed their eyes on the tutor. Others stared at the naked form before them, or at its blank face.

On our table lay an elderly man. His eyes and mouth were closed, his cheeks pronounced, the flesh beneath his chin firm, his hands by his sides, his belly rotund, his knee joints arthritic, his feet wide. Vulnerable and invulnerable. Human and yet not.

We were told when our bodies had died. A whole year ago in my group's case. This man had nobly bequeathed his mortal remains to medical science and apparently we callow students were considered medical science. He had been embalmed very soon after death and had then been immersed in formalin until he was placed on this table. It was a little while before I came to understand that his curious greyness was a feature of the formalin injected to preserve him and not of death itself.

We were not told the names of our bodies or anything personal about them, perhaps to dehumanize them a little. As I now knew *Simpson's Forensic Medicine* almost by heart I might secretly have been hoping for at least a small gunshot wound, but it was explained to us that all the deaths had been from natural causes and that we weren't anyway looking for a cause of death – although we might come across one. This was simply a fundamental introduction to the human body and how it worked. We would be seeing for ourselves how muscle connects to bone, we would be uncovering nerve fibres, examining the plumbing around the kidneys and the vessels around the heart.

We opened our manuals: Aitken, Causey, Joseph and Young's *A Manual of Human Anatomy*, Volume 1, Section 1: Thorax and Upper Limbs. The tutor explained that we would start by cutting straight down the middle of the chest. There was silence as he asked who, in each group, would take up the scalpel. Who was ready to make the first incision into human flesh?

Me, that's who. This was a big test for me. I had to know if I could do it.

I stared at the dead man's face, a blank testament to its owner's long absence. What had he seen? What had he known? He had been a part of the same world as us but in the year since his death that world had changed and moved on and he had not. I looked at his chest. The skin on it was nothing like my skin. It was firm but rubbery.

I picked up the scalpel. I had handled a scalpel before at school but this one felt weighty. How much force would I have to put behind it to cut through human flesh? The eyes of the group were fixed on me. No one spoke.

A hand placed the scalpel on the body's chest. I watched the hand and realized it was mine. The group craned forward. I pressed down. Nothing happened. I pressed harder and felt the skin give. I had made an incision. I pulled the blade slowly, firmly down. The flesh parted cleanly as I cut, in as straight a line as I could, from the jugular notch to the tip of the xiphoid process. We were going to open this flap like opening a book and inside it read the human body! I wanted to dig deeper, right now, and see what was in there.

I was so immersed that I had forgotten the tutor, the other students, the smell of formalin. When the tutor spoke, I looked up, blinking in surprise. Around us, there was movement. At another table, a girl had fainted and was surrounded by a circle of concern. Further down the vast room the swing doors were slamming behind someone's rapid exit. A few more students were heading now towards those doors. One was a friend who was never to return, either to Anatomy classes or medical studies. But among those of us left, there was a new closeness. By dissecting a dead body, we were becoming professionals together. We were joining a very small group, a sect, a tribe. We were initiated. And for me, this maiden flight with the scalpel confirmed my great hope: I belonged here.

As well as Anatomy classes, I was delighted to find that routine post-mortems of patients who had died at University College Hospital were performed daily at lunchtimes and that medical students were invited to view them. And I often did, when a pint of beer and a pie in the Medical Union didn't demand my attention. These teaching examinations were very different from our careful, slow analysis of layer after layer, muscle after muscle, nerve after nerve of the human body. This was a place where I could watch experts at work. They began by slicing down the midline, as I had in Anatomy – but fearlessly. Then I saw them, with great skill, peeling back layers of the body to uncover the organs and the cause of death. That massive cancer, that diseased pancreas, that cerebral haemorrhage, that occluded artery. I wanted to see them all.

University was full of opportunities: to do interesting things, meet people, study, have fun. What a relief it was when I left home to enter this world. Because home had changed. It had become a tense and sometimes comfortless place.

My father, while loving and caring, could also be irascible after my mother's death. Very irascible. I well understand where this came from: his adored partner had died and previously shared burdens all fell on his shoulders. He had been left with a young son at home in need of his love and another son who, feeling his mother's loss acutely, had proved a challenging teenager. On top of it all, my father longed for female company.

Despite his great grief, some time after our mother's death he did start to meet women. Robert and I didn't object: our father was unhappy and one of his early girl-friends, Lillian, was a widow who made him – actually, made all of us – feel much better. She was warm and motherly. She laughed a lot. Our own house was rather quiet, a place of shadows, memories and some empty spaces, while Lillian's was noisy and fun, with good food on the table and friendly guests sitting all around it. And Lillian had parties. Parties! We joined in one Christmas, giggling and fooling with the rest of the guests as an orange was passed down the line from chin to chin.

Unfortunately, Lillian became history. Someone – and the chief suspect was Lillian herself – started a rumour that she and our father were going to marry. He spun on his heel and ran. By then he had turned our mother into something of a saint and perhaps marrying someone else so soon would have felt like less than beatification.

One summer, when we all went on a walking holiday in Devon, our father disappeared, announcing he was look-ing up an old friend. We noticed that he dressed very smartly for this old friend.

The next day he brought the friend to meet us. Her name was Joyce. She had apparently once worked in the same office as our father, but then had left London for reasons unspecified and retreated to her home in the south-west.

Joyce tried hard to be pleasant. She was middle-aged

and nondescript and so sugary sweet to us that she made my toes curl, but I forgave her because I felt rather sorry for her. There was something cowed about Joyce. And indeed, it turned out that she lived with her ill father and her bullying, overbearing mother. Nearby she had a married niece who seemed friendly. Apart from the niece, the inconsequential father and the horrible mother, Joyce was alone in the world.

Her relationship with our father proved to be more than a brief holiday reunion. She began to appear at our home for weekends. She tried to be maternal but she just didn't know how to take charge of teenage boys. On the other hand, she cooked meals, and these were nothing like the meals my father made. Once she even attempted paella, a dish of some daring in the 1960s. She also tidied up and generally brought more of a woman's touch to our male household.

'We don't need a woman's touch,' said Robert. He did not like her saccharine ways and he did not like her inept attempts to fill the gaps. Mother-shaped gaps, gaps where hugs or laughter should be, gaps in the conversation.

I didn't object to her but found myself retreating to friends' houses for much of the time when she came to stay. The fact was, she made our father – well, if not actually happy, then at least less volatile. Because hidden somewhere inside that kind and loving man was a volcano. It could erupt at any time. Suddenly. Unpredictably.

When he lost his temper he screamed, he shouted, he threw things, he terrified me. It didn't happen very often but I always knew the volcano was there, waiting to burst out of him in a red-faced fury, and it was so frightening that once I even wet myself.

We sometimes went to stay near Manchester in the homely, polished house of my maternal grandmother. One morning there, when I was about thirteen, I as usual climbed into bed with my father for a chat and a cup of tea. I was comfortable lolling against his pillows, my body between crisp, linen sheets and a warm mug in my hands, when he suddenly said, 'I'm thinking of marrying Joyce.'

I wanted to shout, 'No!'

I said, 'All right.'

Maybe if he married her he would be happy. And I really did want that. Maybe he would be less prone to mad furies. And I wanted that too.

None of us was invited to the wedding. Our father just drove down to Devon one day and they came back married. For Joyce, it was the escape from her unkind mother that she had dreamed of. Into another kind of jail, maybe, because the running of the house was now placed entirely in her hands. In fact, my father seemed to switch out of domesticity as rapidly as he had once switched into it. Perhaps theirs had been less of a courtship than a job interview. And the job was: housekeeper.

I do believe that Joyce tried to be a good wife. Our home certainly became a feather-duster sort of a place. But for me now there was no escape: Joyce was always there. I couldn't even invite my friends home because she just didn't know how to receive people. But she was kind enough, and, thankfully, she soon abandoned her inept attempts to be a mother to me, perhaps because I made no effort to treat her like one.

My father, Joyce, Robert and I were just four people who happened to live in the same house. Even my father distanced himself from her. I cannot call the marriage a happy one. There would be rows and periods of icy fury. Once, to Robert's and my secret delight, he dumped her with her mother in Devon. But she came back. Then there would be arguments during the day followed by what I realize in retrospect were nocturnal rapprochements. With residual, tooth-grindingly over-loving mornings which didn't, of course, last long. It was frankly baffling.

Robert went to university to study Law, a subject of which our father greatly approved. I missed my brother but at least his absence meant there were fewer arguments and slightly fewer eruptions.

A year later, Robert reappeared, having failed his exams. He announced that he didn't want to study Law anyway. He wanted to study Psychology and Sociology.

Result: exploding father.

'*Sociology?*' he spluttered. 'What kind of a subject is *that*?'

But Robert did study Sociology and then went on to a successful career teaching it at several universities in France. Where he remained for the rest of his working life.

Helen, whenever she visited, would point out all the things that were missing from our home. I chose not to take any notice of my sister but, as I grew older, I could see that she was right. Our mother was being gradually redacted. Over the years, everything associated with her just disappeared until no ornament, picture, photo, piece of darning, sewing basket, book, duster or crockery remained. Poor Joyce might try to replace all these items with something of her own but nothing she bought or did or made could ever fill the void my mother left in that house.

*

By the time I departed for London, then, it sometimes felt as though Joyce had erased my mother and, to some extent, taken my father away too. All that changed when I was a few years into my medical training. He retired from the council and took a job as an accountant in central London. Now our meetings weren't confined to my occasional visits home, with Joyce watching on. We could meet for lunch in town, and we did, often. I had time alone with him again.

We always went to the same restaurant in Greek Street. It was so tiny it sometimes felt like someone's parlour. The food was cheap and delicious and I suspect the kitchens were less than hygienic but it didn't matter: we had warm, close, father–son lunches here. It was like the old days – I mean, before Joyce. He was relaxed and affectionate and so was I, partly because there was no risk of the volcano erupting in a public place.

Maybe he was beginning to see me as a doctor and an adult; anyway, he was expansive. He told me that Joyce's 'niece' was, in fact, her daughter, fathered by a Canadian airman in the war. Joyce's mother had brought the girl up and Joyce was relegated to the role of an occasional aunt – a story certainly not unusual in the 1940s. This great secret shame had enabled Joyce's mother to keep her firmly under the maternal thumb. So, when my father appeared, the middle-aged Joyce saw him as her escape route.

It was easy now to understand why she had been unable to show the slightest motherly feeling towards two teenage boys. She had never been given a chance to mother her own child.

My father even described the misery of his wedding to

her and how, driving down to Devon for it, he had seriously considered crashing the car. Not badly enough to kill himself, just enough to evade the marriage. But, typically of him, he had decided he had better go through with it in case Joyce – or more likely her mother – sued him for breach of promise.

I smiled at the way my father tried to be correct in everything he did, and remembered the dictionary he had given me when I was sixteen. In the front he had laboriously written, in a perfect copperplate hand, set inside a box carefully drawn in ink, some lines from Alexander Pope. What were those lines? I had learned them by heart as a teenager but now I could capture only a fragment.

In all you speak, let Truth and Candour shine . . .

I determined to go back to my flat and relearn all the lines. I remembered that the poem offered a code for proper living and correct behaviour. My father believed in that code and wanted me to believe in it too.

At one of those lunches he told me how, after my mother's death, he had many times come close to committing suicide. Only the feeling that he could not leave Robert and me stopped him. To cope, he was prescribed Valium. Gradually he weaned himself off it by substituting alcohol to help him sleep and relax. I never saw him drunk: he just had at the most a pint or two of Devon cider each evening, but that seemed to make his loss and his late, unhappy marriage more bearable.

And as well as talking openly about his own life, including his regrets and mistakes, he told me how proud he was of the three of us: Helen the teacher, Robert the university lecturer and me the doctor. And how proud our mother would have been. I was deeply moved to receive this blessing, which really felt as though it came from both parents. Even now, although my mother and father are long dead, I can allow myself to feel touched by those words, delivered in a shabby little restaurant in Soho. How lucky I was to have those adult, honest conversations with that dear man.

After a year, they ended. My father was offered a lectureship in the Department of Management at Loughborough University. This was quite an achievement for someone who had left school at fourteen. He and Joyce now had to sell the family home and move to another part of the country. I did wonder what effect this would have on them but in fact it improved their relationship considerably: no tragic first wife had left indelible fingerprints in their Loughborough house.

Most students returned to their family home for the holidays but this was a habit I kicked early. Summer holidays were spent working and travelling. In 1974, driving up the coast of Italy towards Venice in a Ford Anglia with my mates, blissfully unaware of the political upheavals we had just left behind us in Greece, *Tubular Bells* on the cassette player . . . well, it didn't matter that home wasn't there for me now that my father and Joyce had moved away. One taproot of my life had shifted just as other roots were forming. I had a new girlfriend and she seemed more like the future.

# 6

I was almost thirty before I performed my first post-mortem. There had been the usual house jobs in different departments around the hospital, from surgery to gynae-cology, from dermatology to psychiatry. Only when these were completed as 1980 ended did I begin to focus on my goal. It was more than ten years since I'd started medical school and I hadn't even reached the first rung of the ladder to becoming a forensic pathologist, which was to qualify as a histo- (or hospital) pathologist.

In general, pathology is a science that enables us to understand disease by studying it in micro-detail: we name it, find how it is caused, learn how it progresses. Everyone has some sort of contact with a path lab without really being aware of it: all urine and blood samples are sent there, for instance. Of course, staring at so many samples in such minute detail is not glamorous work and, unsurprisingly, the pathology department is always somewhere at the back of the hospital, far away from patients.

Qualifying as a hospital pathologist involves spending a huge amount of time looking at microscope slides, studying both normal and diseased tissue. I have lost count of the hours I spent peering at, for instance, cancerous cells.

I found all this very tedious because I knew that, when I actually reached my goal and became a forensic pathologist,

I'd be referring such slides to specialists and seldom looking at them myself. But I had to study this now. There are many pathologists who will carry out post-mortems, if death is believed to have occurred naturally, to establish the exact cause and this would be the next part of my training – because how could I examine suspicious, unexplained deaths and view them forensically if I couldn't recognize natural causes?

So, there was nothing of the criminal in my first post-mortem. The patient had died at St George's, Tooting, and the case had been chosen specially for me because it was considered straightforward.

I knew I would be surrounded by senior colleagues and helpful mortuary staff but nevertheless the butterflies in my stomach as I went to work reminded me of my first day at school. Handfuls of rain banged against the bus windows and then ran down them, blurring the world outside, and I longed for the day when I could afford a good pair of shoes which would keep my feet dry and a good coat to keep me warm. I sat huddled upstairs at the front of the bus as it rattled and swayed to Tooting Broadway. I tried to distract myself by rereading, yet again, the medical notes of the deceased. I'd been given them the day before, discussed them with the more senior trainees and almost knew them by heart already.

I had watched quite a few post-mortems at the mortuary and had half anticipated, half dreaded the time when it would be my turn to take up the scalpel here. Like the first Anatomy class, it was a test – no fainting, blanching or vomiting allowed. Not because this would mean the end of my career, but because I knew my colleagues would

47

never let me forget it. The same was true of mistakes. The others would correct me – and then tease me about it endlessly. And I really did want to do well. No cutting my fingers instead of the patient, no making holes in critical organs, no slicing the bowel by mistake. I wanted clean cuts, decisive exposure of the relevant organs, correct note-taking, accurate diagnosis. Plus, a bit of luck. Oh, and a lot of courage.

Most people recoil at the smell of the mortuary. I'd say now that mortuaries don't smell at all, but it may be that I'm just used to it. Certainly, in those days it seemed to me that the nose was assaulted by the whiff of formalin, a smell as acrid as broken branches: perhaps holly in winter or an elder bush snapped in summer. But far more penetrating.

The first sound heard on entering a mortuary is the rise and fall of almost unfailingly friendly voices. And, believe it or not, often those voices may be laughing, as in any office or workplace in the land. In fact, if undertakers are coming and going, I think the word is banter, although I have never heard jokes at the expense of the dead. In my experience, they are always treated with the greatest respect.

The dead's entrance is unseen by the public. It is usually next to a neat, bright office where arrivals are carefully, no, meticulously booked in and then taken down well-lit corridors to the banks of fridges, ten or fifteen of them, in a solid line.

The fridges are a few metres high. Inside, each has shelving for about six bodies. The dead slide on their trays from their metal trolleys onto their shelf. *Clang*. The door is shut. *Whoomp*. The trolley is parked, ready for its next use. *Clatter*. That is the sound of the mortuary. *Clang, whoomp, clatter*.

I already knew these sounds and smells well. In fact, mortuaries were just beginning to feel like home. But I can't pretend that today this familiarity brought any comfort.

'Cup of tea, Dick?' offered a kind assistant. I couldn't even answer him, let alone drink it.

The other mortuary staff were determined to treat my rite of passage as a joke.

'Er, Dick, make sure you get the right body, would you?'

Etc., etc. I tried to laugh but risus sardonicus – the grim, fixed smile of strychnine poisoning – seemed to have set in.

I emerged from the changing room in my scrubs and found mortuary wellies. They were a deathly white, which, that day, perfectly matched my face. I wore a pair of bright yellow Marigold gloves and an apron. The kit has changed a lot over the years but then the apron was something akin to the aprons worn in abattoirs and butchers' shops. The gloves were no doubt cheap and good for washing dishes, but they protected you only from germs, not cuts.

'And, remember, Dick, those gloves also show you where your fingers are . . .' were the final words of helpful advice from the staff as I passed the fridges and entered the post-mortem room.

The patient was a middle-aged woman who had been admitted to the hospital with severe chest pains and had then died on the coronary care unit some days later. The mortuary staff had her waiting for me on a porcelain table.

She was still wearing her shroud. Wrapping bodies really neatly in tight sheets used to be one of the great nursing skills, like making a bed with hospital corners, but it is seldom if ever seen now. It gave respect to the dead but exasperated the nurses: it could take them an hour or so to shroud a body well, only for us to simply pull the sheet off in the mortuary to perform the post-mortem. No wonder busy ward staff abandoned all that linen origami and started using simple paper shrouds instead.

The mortuary staff removed the shroud to reveal the body.

I stared at her. Anatomy dissection had been one thing, with its dead bodies so long pickled and grey that it was possible to forget they had ever been alive at all. But this was quite another thing. Here was a fresh body. Here was a woman who, within the last twenty-four hours, was living and breathing and talking to her family and to her doctors. According to her notes, she had said she was determined to get better and go to her granddaughter's wedding in a month's time. And then was dead within the hour.

In fact, she looked really rather healthy and not very dead at all. I had the uncanny feeling that she might wake up at any moment. And I was going to cut into her pink flesh. Run a knife right down her torso and then open her. Surgeons, of course, do just that, but for surgeons there's a good reason, at least in theory: they are trying to save a life or improve its quality. I could make no such claim. At that moment, I wondered if I didn't have more in common with a homicidal maniac than a doctor.

My older colleagues stopped joshing and watched me

closely as I carried out my external examination of the body, looking for marks and any indications of the cause of death.

I'd always wanted to do this. I'd worked hard to arrive at this point. But now, suddenly, my ambition to become Keith Simpson and specialize in forensic pathology to help solve crimes seemed a schoolboy fantasy. The woman lying motionless on the porcelain table in front of me was the reality. Whatever had possessed me? I must have been insane to want to do this.

'OK?' asked a voice. Humour had been replaced by concern.

I took a deep breath, steeled myself, picked up the knife and placed it at the little notch in the centre of the base of her neck between the inner ends of the collar bones. Her skin did not resist as I pushed on the blade. I pulled it through the midline. Firmly because I was trying to stop my hand from shaking. Down, down, right down the body to the pubic bone.

My second cut along the same line took me through a layer of bright yellow fat. The patient was overweight. Fat solidifies and becomes more fixed to the skin once the body has cooled down in death and it can simply be peeled away. Underneath is the muscle layer and beneath that is the ribcage of the thin person who is always there inside that round body – but hidden.

My next cut was also easy, the cut through muscle. It is hard to believe how much like the carcases hanging at the butcher's the human body looks when stripped down to the bone, and how like a steak human muscle can appear.

Now I could fold the skin sideways and outwards from

the midline, as though opening a book. Even with a breast each side, this is easy. The main problem was to make sure my knife didn't cut through the thin skin around the neck: if her relatives paying their last respects saw this, it would look shocking to them, like a stabbing. In fact, mortuary staff are highly skilled at repairing the mistakes of junior doctors – but it would cost me a bottle of whisky, something I could ill afford.

Once the skin, fat and muscle are pulled back it is easy to cut through and then remove the front of the ribs. And when I had done this, there before me were this woman's internal organs laid out for my inspection.

Her lungs looked purple and swollen. They were flecked with soot.

'Hmm, looks like a smoker,' said my older colleagues, shaking their heads in disapproval. While they hid their nicotine-stained fingers.

'But the purple colour suggests oedema,' added one.

'Pulmonary oedema . . .' I echoed nervously. That meant the lungs had become waterlogged with fluid. This can happen when the heart is failing from disease but I knew it very often happens during the actual process of dying as the heart finally fails. Since death can be caused for one of a thousand reasons, waterlogged lungs alone are not usually helpful for diagnostic purposes.

I opened the sac inside which the heart nestles. It is just to the left side of the chest.

'No blood or excess fluid. But it looks like she's had a massive infarct,' I said quickly, before anyone could tell me. About a third of the muscle at the front of the heart was distinctly paler than the rest, indicating that it had been deprived of its blood supply and oxygen. A myocardial infarct, colloquially called a heart attack, is the death of heart muscle: if the patient survives the initial damage then eventually the muscle becomes scarred. But this heart attack was too recent for scarring.

'What was her blood pressure the last time it was taken?' they asked me.

'High. 180/100.'

'High blood pressure . . . oh, and she was such a big-hearted woman,' hinted the others.

It looked like a normal heart to me.

'Is it enlarged?'

'Wall of the left ventricle seems a bit thick . . . weigh it.'

The heart weighed 510g. That's huge.

They said, 'What do you think?'

'Um . . . lungs full of fluid. High blood pressure, left ventricle enlarged and an infarct. One of the coronary arteries is blocked by thrombus.'

'Yes. But which one?'

Back to Anatomy class. The anatomy of the heart. For my own personal reasons, I'd spent a lot of time studying this organ. Its structure. Its pathology. Its associated pathogenic mechanisms. Its arteries. Its valves. Especially the mitral. Yes, I knew about hearts.

'There should be a blockage in . . . er . . . the left anterior descending artery?'

They nodded. 'Take a look!'

I did, and there it was. A big, red, solid clot that had halted blood flow along the artery, depriving the heart muscle of the blood and oxygen it needed. And so, it had simply died.

What a remarkable mechanism the human seemed to me that day. As my fear drained away I became absorbed in my work. But I still had time to experience that sense of wonder at the body: its intricate systems, its colours and, yes, its beauty. For blood is not just red – it is bright red. The gall bladder is not just green, it is the green of jungle foliage. The brain is white and grey – and that is not the grey of a November sky, it is the silver-grey of darting fish. The liver is not a dull school-uniform brown, it is the sharp red-brown of a freshly ploughed field.

When I had finished examining each organ and they had all been replaced in the body, the mortuary staff moved in to work their magic of reconstruction.

'Well done,' one of the senior trainees said. 'Wasn't so bad, was it?'

It was over and I had been slow – it was well past lunchtime – but I had done all right. I had put my feelings about older women with heart problems to one side and had recalled my training and then conducted myself in an entirely clinical way. As I washed afterwards I felt flushed with relief. I was a horse that, after racing round the track for years and years, had been nervous about facing a hurdle – and then had easily cleared it.

The post-mortem turned out not to be the hardest job that day. Meeting the deceased woman's relatives was far more demanding. Given a choice, I would have preferred not to see them at all. But they had sensibly asked for a meeting with the pathologist to help them understand why she had died. And that pathologist was evidently me.

I was saved by my colleagues, who did all the talking. I was simply not up to the task, so unbearable did I find the relatives' shock and grief. In fact, I felt utterly helpless in the face of their emotion. Their misery seemed to transmit itself to me, to my mind and my body, as if we were attached by invisible wires. I don't remember if I said anything at all: if I did, I probably just kept repeating how very sorry I was for their loss. Mostly I am sure I nodded while my colleagues talked.

The meeting introduced me – or, perhaps no introduction was necessary – to the awful collision between the silent, unfeeling dead and immensity of feeling they generate in the living. I left the room with relief, making a mental note to avoid the bereaved at all costs and stick to the safe world inhabited by the dead, with its facts, its measurements, its certainties. In their universe, there was a complete absence of emotion. Not to mention its ugly sister, pain.

# 7

Even at thirty, I was much better at managing strong emotion than experiencing it. I suppose that in my boyhood I must have learned to work hard at suppressing the anxiety caused by my mother's illness. And then at just carrying on, despite my grief at her loss. Our home, with its silences and spaces, became a sort of desert where, to my relief, strong emotion did not flourish. Although from time to time it would appear so suddenly through my brother's challenges or my father's vaporizing tempers that it seemed to be something very scary, dropped suddenly from another planet. It was certainly very hard to believe it had been there, beneath the surface, all along.

I would have liked life to be emotionally uneventful but by the time I performed my first post-mortem that was certainly not the case. I returned home from the mortuary and opened the front door to hear the wails of my new baby son. He was oblivious to the extraordinarily powerful love and bewilderment he stirred in his parents. And as for my wife, she showed no sign of satisfaction with the flat emotional landscape I preferred.

Jen and I had met at the hospital when I was a student. She was the beautiful, dark-haired nurse who mopped my brow during finals, who entered my life with a great vitality and whose cleverness I admired. Each day she finished most of the *Times* crossword at ridiculous speed – although not quite as quickly as her father, Austin, could finish the *Telegraph*'s. He had retired from a distinguished career in the Colonial Police in Uganda after seeing service in the Indian Mounted Police and was now living on the Isle of Man.

Jen's parents were the beating heart of Manx society. When she took me home for the first time I was overwhelmed by her dizzy, busy and, it seemed to me, luxurious world. Austin presided with great charm over a living room full of visitors. Whisky and sodas, noise and laughter, the great old house's lack of physical warmth was unnoticeable for the warmth of the welcome there. The furniture and curtains were all swathes and swags. The immense, if slightly dilapidated, kitchen smelled good. And there were always two dogs asleep in front of the oven.

It didn't matter if we arrived late at night; Jen's mother, Maggie, gin-and-tonic at a precarious angle in one hand, wooden spoon waving in the other, would greet us extravagantly and ply us with fine food. She was the sort of woman whose presence defined any party. The sort of parent my siblings assured me my own mother had once been, although I could hardly imagine such a thing. Viewed from the noisy whirl of Austin and Maggie's home on the Isle of Man, the house of my upbringing seemed a sparse, silent place. Empty, even. I tried to remember with affection the radiogram, the antimacassars, the swirly carpet in my childhood home. And couldn't.

On our marriage, Jen's kind parents helped us buy our new home in Surrey. I had qualified as a doctor, finished my 'house' jobs and was just about to start training as a pathologist. Jen was now working as a health visitor. We couldn't, for a while, afford a proper bed or any furniture at all, but we were happy. Then, after a few years, we knew that the time was right to start a family.

We were unaccustomed to adversity but here it came, making up for lost time. Jen had a miscarriage. We were both devastated. I had no idea how to deal with my overwhelming feelings of loss, my sense of the child that could have been, the life that might have been lived, nor what to do with the love that should have belonged to that baby. My pain was an enormous, invisible thing I carried awkwardly around. Where on earth was I to put it? This was so preoccupying that I was entirely incapable of offering Jen enough support in her own great sadness. Was I supposed to say something? Do something? If so, what?

I failed to say it, whatever it was, I failed to do it, whatever it was, and I also failed to admit that I was completely out of my emotional depth. So, when we lost the next baby, then the next, I became more and more distressed by Jen's apparently unassuageable grief. It was a true reflection of my own unexpressed devastation but, rather than look at it, I confess, with many regrets, that I turned my back. I became increasingly isolated. So did she.

I did manage to tell her how much I loved her and how sad and confused I was that our babies could not seem to grow larger than a cluster of cells. Would that do?

No. She seemed to expect more from me. And she was right. Although I still couldn't imagine what I was supposed to offer. Just as, when a young boy, I didn't really know what people had wanted me to do after my mother's death.

Finally, when she found she was carrying yet another baby, Jen was confined for almost the entire pregnancy to bed rest in hospital. It was not a happy time, separating and isolating us from each other still further. Until, at full-term, a beautiful boy, whom we named Christopher, was born one winter's day.

Most parents will remember the chaos of their first, longed-for arrival. I'd been overwhelmed because there was no baby. Now I was overwhelmed because there was a baby. And so was Jen, even though she was by now an experienced health visitor. As for me, I was a doctor with a stint in paediatrics behind me. But we were both taken aback by the weeping, the sheer dissatisfaction with which our little prince responded to our efforts to please him. And all the time we were awash with a love for him which was so deep and passionate it shook me to the core. And his apparent lack of appreciation of our efforts perhaps shocked us both.

When I returned home after completing my first post-mortem and opened the door to Chris's familiar, high-pitched wail and the sweet smell of baby oil, I found Jen upstairs. The busy mother of our tiny son was elbow-deep in baths and nappies, gently shushing the eternally protesting Chris. Downstairs, her books were propped open in the living room: she'd just started studying for an Open University degree but Chris and his yells had seen off that plan this evening.

Every moment of Jen's time was filled: no wonder she had forgotten it was such a big day for me. And now that the hurdle of my first post-mortem was receding into the distance, this racehorse began to wonder if the hurdle had really been so high anyway.

I went upstairs to see them both. Chris looked at me and wrinkled his face into a ball from which a smile might have emerged. Or a roar of disapproval. Predictably, it was a roar. I took him from Jen and he wailed some more. I rocked him, swung him, gazed at him, pulled faces at him. His tiny features twisted themselves again into a comical but unbecoming ball. A smile? Of course not. Out came another huge wail. How, how to stop him?

Jen put the baby to bed while I made the evening meal. Miraculously, Chris's roars upstairs subsided just as the meal was ready downstairs. We ate it, relishing the silence as much as the food. After supper, we both studied. I was in a world of exams without end, a world Jen, on her degree course, was just entering.

And now it's late. I am exhausted, having spent much of last night worrying about and preparing for today's post-mortem. The day is over and when my head hits the pillow I know all I want is sleep, sweet sleep. I can feel it engulfing me. My body relaxes happily, I am slipping downstream when suddenly . . . *Waaaaah!*

Chris. Again. God, again. He cries so much that we're starting to suspect that, despite being breast-fed, he might have a lactose intolerance. But what good are all the theories in the world going to do me now? Because Chris may be allergic to milk but he has excellent lungs and he is crying and one of us will have to do something.

'Your turn,' mumbles Jen.

I get up. The house is still and cold.

I reach into the cot and scoop up Chris's hot, stiff, angry little body. I love him but I want to go back to sleep. I walk around the house, cradling him in my arms. Lack of sleep is depriving me of my humanity, I am a robot doomed to walk until the end of time with my kicking little bundle. I know the bundle is a baby, a vulnerable baby. But I am beginning to wonder. Is he, in fact, a tyrant? A tyrant whose sole and monstrous aim it is to deprive me of what I crave most, sweet sleep?

Gradually, after a long, long time, gentle rocking persuades him to cry less, to yawn more, to close his eyes. I listen to his breathing. Even. Deep. Yes, he is asleep.

Very, very gently, stealthily, like an art thief, I traipse to the nursery and place my tiny masterpiece oh so gently into his cot. I pull the blankets over his sweet-smelling body. He is pliable now with drowsiness. I watch him for a moment. He pulls a face and that may mean . . . I hold my breath but all remains silent. He is dreaming. I feel something similar to joy as I creep towards our bed. The duvet closes over me like an embrace, I shut my eyes. And then . . . *Waaaaaah!*

What desperate parent hasn't feared that he might shake the baby or lose his temper and chuck the baby into the cot, or give the baby a short, sharp slap to stop the noise? What desperate parent hasn't been terrified by his own pressing need for respite from the constant demands, the wearing, piercing *Waaaaah*?

I knew that, although Chris was distressed, he was safe enough. I knew I needed a few quiet moments. I shut the bedroom door on my crying son and went downstairs into the kitchen. I shut this door behind me too. He was still crying but the crying was distant. I covered my ears. I could no longer hear him. I continued to cover my ears for five minutes. Breathing deeply. Regaining my equilibrium. Then I returned to his cot. Maybe not full to the brim with love, but certainly lovingly, and with my compassion rekindled. I rocked him gently back to sleep.

After that, we researched neo-natal milk allergy and Jen stopped eating and drinking dairy products. Chris became almost immediately a different child. He slept. He even smiled. But I am grateful for all I learned from that wailing baby. Thank you, Chris, for giving me this understanding of the great pressure some parents face.

# 8

Two years later, we had another child, Anna. She was lactose-tolerant and a much easier baby; or maybe it was we, her parents, who were easier now we had some experience.

By the time Anna was born, my first post-mortem was far behind me and so were many more. As soon as I'd passed the initial part of my specialist pathology exams, I gathered speed, understanding and skill by working in mortuaries throughout London, from Wembley to Finchley to Tooting.

I'd arrive for a morning's work to find the dead waiting patiently for me on a line of tables. These were not suspicious deaths. Most were believed to have died of natural causes, which it was my job to ascertain.

Many such causes are immediately obvious. Something looking like a blob of redcurrant jelly in the brain? That's a stroke. Severe heart disease? That one is rapidly settled by dissection of the coronary arteries to find them crackly with plaque, or opening up the heart sac to discover a blocked valve or the soft shadow of oxygen-starved heart muscle. You can see and assess the kidneys quite quickly, also the lungs, spleen, liver, biliary tree, gall bladder, pancreas, stomach and bowel. The heart does take a bit longer and so do the throat, neck, trachea and bronchi.

This was a time of great change for those of us carrying out post-mortems. The average length of time it took my predecessors, including my hero Professor Simpson, to carry out one post-mortem and ascertain cause of death where no crime was suspected might shock today's pathologists: often just fifteen minutes. That was partly because mortuary staff saved time by preparing the bodies and removing the internal organs for examination even before the pathologist arrived. That practice was still the norm when I started. It had also been usual – and still was in places – once the cause of death had been found, to move on to the next patient with only a brief recording of the rest of the organs. Old-school pathologists argued that when there was clearly a heart problem, there was no need to waste time weighing the kidneys. And the coroners' own pro-forma report, published by the government, seemed to confirm this, because it was just one page long.

Of course, this led to whispered tales of pathologists who just looked at the heart and, if they found it at all diseased, declared heart disease the cause of death, bothering to look no further and ignoring the fact that most people in the Western world have some degree of atheroma (furred-up arteries) and many may be walking around with that same degree of heart disease. No one knew how many quick-fire pathologists were practising, but there was a strong suspicion that their excessive diagnoses of heart disease distorted government cause-of-death statistics.

Those days had all but passed before I became fully established. It wasn't just that I had been trained to examine bodies more thoroughly, but also because inside me there was always a forensic pathologist bursting to get out. I was keen and curious to see if a death was more suspicious than it at first appeared. I was also anxious to establish not just the immediate cause of death but anything relative to it.

But how hard it was for keen, young Dr Shepherd to push in the old public mortuaries for the newfangled practices he had been taught. These included external examination of a body before it is touched by mortuary staff, weighing and study of each organ, samples taken for toxicology or histology, detailed recording of findings . . . even just brighter lights. The staff didn't like any of this. Their mortuaries were often set at the back of some dark cemetery, and the elderly staff had worked there for years and were used to the old ways of carrying out postmortems. I didn't have to listen very hard to hear mutinous mutterings wafting from their offices about 'new boys' and 'the good old days'. Sometimes, if I insisted on showing a particular interest in a case they considered routine, they got really annoyed and denied me my cup of tea. A cruel punishment which seldom lasted long.

I did, however, learn something from the old-school thinking. Those charlatans who were only too ready to name the first irregularity they encountered as cause of death introduced young Dr Shepherd to truth's elasticity. Truth is based upon knowledge. So, of course, it can be compromised by incomplete knowledge. As a doctor I sought truth through facts. As a pathologist I was now learning that truth could be directly affected by choices I made, by how many facts I chose to study. It was the first step in what was to become a lifelong examination of the nature of truth.

Carrying out large numbers of post-mortems as scrupulously as I could, and always on the look-out for homicide,

I came to know the human body and its many weaknesses as well as I knew the Tube map – better, perhaps. In those years, I was constantly busy: studying, teaching medical students and, of course, performing post-mortems. Death had become a way of life, and in the next phase of my training I had to be more or less dragged out of mortuaries to spend more time staring at those dreaded microscope slides of human disease.

Disconsolate, I sneaked away from the hospital path labs whenever I could to sit in the office of my great friend and mentor, the forensic pathologist Dr Rufus Crompton. He had helped pilot my career and now he let me study piles of police photos, read reports and immerse myself in all things forensic: scenes, injuries, excuses and explanations of the accused, witness statements, everything. Just to remind myself what lay waiting for me when I no longer had to stare at end-to-end disease slides. And, eventually, I did begin to carry out, under supervision, post-mortems on sudden or suspicious deaths, the sort of deaths coroners would open inquests for and the police would investigate.

At last, sixteen years after I started my medical training, my son now aged six and my daughter four, I qualified. I was a forensic pathologist. That goal I had fixed on since encountering Simpson's book as a teenager had been achieved. But of course, it was only the beginning.

I landed my first job at Guy's Hospital. My boss was to be Iain West, the man who was top dog in our profession. After any homicide or disaster, his department was the go-to place for the police, coroners or solicitors. And, even more exciting, this was the very place where my hero, Professor Keith Simpson, had worked.

There were four pathologists, and we were always technically 'on call' – but we could pass the work round among ourselves. Less interesting cases, that is, those which were medically or forensically straightforward, usually went down the pecking order. And as the newly qualified arrival, I was at the bottom of that order.

When there was no homicide to examine we were teaching and lecturing to medical students or more professional audiences such as police or coroners' officers. The students were mostly in the fourth year of their general medical training and, for many of them, this was their introduction to a world their comfortable homes had not exposed them to before. Rapes, murders, assaults; they lapped it up and the lecture hall overflowed. There were students sitting in the aisles and standing at the back. They learned not just about life but about how stupidity and inhumanity leads to fatal injury, and I hope they learned a little about recognizing when a death is suspicious.

It was a pleasure to hold forth to enraptured rooms, but we spent a great deal less time lecturing about homicide than we did looking at it. Because London seemed to be awash with murder, or at least sudden and suspicious deaths. We had meetings in our offices, poring over photos, arguing about cases, and then we continued the discussions in the pub, sometimes with barristers or the police. The place just buzzed.

Of course, I treated my earliest cases, simple though they were, with great concentration and seriousness, working with guidance from Iain and other colleagues.

But the day had to come when I went out alone to my first homicide as a lecturer in forensic medicine at Guy's and, because we were so busy, it came quickly. It is hard to describe how proud I felt as I headed towards a dull block of flats in Croydon where a body awaited me. Proud, and not a little nervous.

It was a weekday, mid-morning. My heart was beating hard, perhaps with the effort of trying to look like a pathologist who had been called out many times before.

Ringed by a physical and human barrier of tape and police officers, and beyond them press and neighbours, a young white man lay in a roadside gutter. A Metropolitan Police photographer was already busy but paused as I bent to examine the body.

The deceased was lying on his back and nothing more serious than a few cuts and abrasions were visible on his face. But I knew a lot more was happening than that because beneath his upper body was a pool of blood.

I reached out. He still felt warm to my touch. He was not yet stiff, although his muscles were already tightening, most notably around the neck and jaw and in the fingers.

I rolled him over. His thick jacket had a stab hole at the back. That's where all the blood had come from. I let his body return to its original position.

As the photographer worked I made more notes for my post-mortem report. In it I would have to describe the scene and what I had found there, then I would give details of my full examination of the body at the mortuary, and finally a conclusion about the cause of death. The last part would, hopefully, be straightforward, since there was still blood dripping from the stab hole in the young man's back. But there was a lot of work to do between now and my final conclusions.

The victim had not yet been identified, so for now he was simply recorded as Unknown Young Caucasian Male. He looked about eighteen. He was slim and some might describe him as handsome. I made a diagram of what I saw, especially noting the position of bloodstains in the road and on the adjacent pavement. I also scribbled notes about the scene, the deceased's clothes and the position of the body. The notes were to re-emerge later in the post-mortem report as:

> Rigor mortis was established around the neck and jaw but was less marked elsewhere on the body. These findings are consistent with death occurring about 3 hours earlier.

Still trying to sound authoritative, and not as though this was my first case, I asked the coroner's officer to have the body removed to the mortuary. I followed it there, where I was joined by various police officers, including a detective superintendent. I read this in my report now with incredulity. There is no way a 'super' would turn out today for a street stabbing.

At the mortuary there were further photographs, and I wrote detailed notes about the victim's clothes before I even started on his body.

> Jacket: heavy blood staining on the left side of the back. Gravel from roadway also present. Three defects in the fabric. Defect one – 8cm to the left of the midline seam,

approx 21cm from the collar. 8mm in length, approx horizontal. Defect two – 12cm right of midline seam, approx. 21cm from collar. 16mm length. Vertical. Defect three – 3.5cm below the same approximately on the lateral midline of the right sleeve. 18mm in length. Horizontal.

Sports shirt: blood staining on the back and left side. Three defects in the fabric . . .

Blood staining on the back of the waistband of the jeans, boxer shorts and underpants. Blood splashes noted on the back of the lower half of the legs of the jeans . . .

When I had scribbled several pages about the clothes, we removed them, putting each one in a separate evidence bag, which was taken and labelled by a police officer.

Once the patient lay naked on the table for post-mortem, I could see how extensive his wounds were. Three stab wounds in his back, one of which had clearly been the fatal wound, and nine additional significant injuries to the abdomen and face. In my notes are body charts – blank outlines of bodies – and on these I drew details of the injuries, numbering them, and then wrote notes:

Five injuries to left side of face:
  (i) 3mm diameter contusion immediately above lateral margin of left eyebrow.
  (ii) 10mm curved laceration with associated bruising on lateral margin of left upper eyelid.
  (iii) 20 × 22mm abrasion over lateral aspect of left zygomatic arch. Surface dried . . .

Lacerations are different from the clean incisions of knife wounds. In a laceration, the skin is torn apart rather than sliced and this is caused by a blunt weapon. Not many people regard a road or a kerb or a building as a 'weapon', but if a body slams against it, then its effect is that of a weapon. In this case, I thought laceration could have been caused by the victim's head hitting the kerb when he fell.

Abrasions are scratches or grazes, which seldom penetrate below the epidermis – the skin's outer hard layer. They don't, therefore, actually bleed, but they can ooze blood, often as spots. They can be a feature of road traffic accidents because they are caused by sliding over rough surfaces. Of course, grazes are very common in life, but forensically they are interesting because they can also occur after death. Supposing the young man's body had been dragged along the road: this might have caused the abrasions but it could be difficult to tell from them if he had been dragged before or after he was murdered.

Contusions are bruises. Damage to the small veins and arteries causes them to break and bleed. Children have more resilient tissues so their skin can bruise less easily than the skin of older people which has lost its elasticity. Bruises can be deceptive, however, because their major component is blood, and this is both fluid and biodegradable. Result: bruises change over time and under the influence of gravity. Most notably, they change colour. That is because, once blood is outside the confines of a blood vessel, the body starts to break it down. Generally speaking, bruises go from purple to yellow to green to brown. There has been much research into dating a bruise from its colour and it would be very useful if any of the systems devised to do this were reliable; unfortunately, none is.

It can certainly be disconcerting to find that bruises become more prominent after death and even that 'new' bruises have appeared days or even weeks later. This doesn't mean the body has been injured at the mortuary. It is simply a sign that red blood cells have continued to leak from the damaged blood vessels – although pulled by gravity rather than pushed by blood pressure.

It took a long time to write all the notes on the victim's exterior injuries. When I had finished I looked up, blinking. The police officers blinked back at me. There was a pause while I remembered what to do next.

These days I wouldn't experience the slightest shame in pausing to think but then I so wanted to appear entirely in control that I had to pretend to scribble notes for a moment to buy myself time. I wished the staff would turn off Radio 1 but was too shy to ask them.

Chris de Burgh was singing about a lady in red.

I tried to concentrate. Of course. Swabs next. Of the genitalia, anus and mouth so the scientists could look for signs of a sexual assault.

'Any chance you could switch that racket off?' said the super.

The staff weren't very pleased; however, they did so, to my relief. But now the room seemed eerily silent as I took samples of the young man's hair as well as clippings from his nails, which could be searched for skin or fibres or any other debris trapped there that might link him to an assailant or a place. At the end of the post-mortem, I would take samples of blood, urine, tissues for histology and anything else that might be relevant.

The exhibits were all marked with my initials and a number (RTS/1). I wrote each label with a new boy's pride. For thirty years that unique triplet of letters has signified my involvement in a case but on that day, the first time I wrote them, the letters looked stark and new, like a school uniform at the beginning of term.

Everyone in the room – the coroner's officer and the police officers – waited for me to start the internal examination. It is a little-known duty of police officers to observe post-mortems: their presence is an important part of the protocol. The super had, of course, seen quite a few in his time, but for the young PC who also witnessed the process it was a first. He had been looking distinctly miserable during the external examination and when I picked up my scalpel he turned deathly pale.

'All right, lad?' asked the super.

The constable nodded grimly.

I tried to think of something to say to make him feel better. But I couldn't. I was too busy trying to look as if I had performed plenty of forensic post-mortems entirely alone.

'Oh, you'll soon get used to it,' I said airily, to hide my own nerves.

The PC swallowed. I attempted a reassuring smile but was so anxious that my muscles felt oddly stiff and the smile may have been more of a grimace because the PC did not return it but instead looked alarmed. Then, as I opened the body, I became aware that the young officer did not take his eyes off me. The way he stared at my face was so disconcerting that a couple of my cuts wobbled slightly. I glanced up at him and saw that he wore the fixed mask of sheer terror. Staring at my face was apparently his method of not looking at what my hands were doing.

I would have liked to find a way to reassure and support him. But I was so tense that I was without the resources to help. Even the experienced super and the coroner's officer, who had greeted each other like the veterans of many cases together, had now stopped talking and were watching me in deep silence. Usually the mortuary staff can be counted on to lighten the atmosphere with a quip or a comment but today they were oddly still. Why didn't someone talk? Just say something? No one did. I even found myself wishing they would switch on the radio again. Although perhaps to a different station.

They watched as I tracked the wounds internally. When I examined the victim's facial wounds from the inside, the PC's body shook suddenly and he rushed from the room, hand over his mouth.

'Oh-oh,' said the super. The coroner's officer laughed. Then we reverted to silence.

I carried out a routine dissection of the victim's internal systems and organs and checked that there were no rib or other fractures. It is essential to make sure there is no contributing natural cause of death. But the young man proved to be in perfect health. Apart, of course, from the fact that he was dead.

I was glad when the post-mortem ended and asked myself why the atmosphere had been so unlike other forensic post-mortems I had attended. I won't say they are usually jolly affairs but there is a camaraderie, or anyway a

74

level of noise or discussion, which was completely absent today. What could the problem be?

Back at the office I started to write my report.

Stab wound 1 lay 6cm to the left of the midline on the back ... the upper margin of the wound was sharply pointed: the lower margin was blunted ... the wound measured 26mm in length ... The track of the wound passed between the fifth and sixth ribs of the left hemithorax ... the track then entered the left upper lobe on its posterior aspect and passed forwards, slightly downwards and towards the midline. The track transversed the upper lobe of the left lung and incised the left pulmonary artery ... This incision was 40mm in length and irregular ... Over 1 litre of partly clotted blood was present in the left hemithorax ... There was no bruising of the skin adjacent to the wound.

So, on the inside of the body, the wound was almost twice as long as it was externally. I included some analysis.

The route of the track through the muscles of the back was such that the left arm must have been raised at the time of the injury. The discrepancy between the size of the internal and external injuries suggests movement while the weapon was within the chest cavity.

This movement of the knife could have been significant. It certainly indicated that here was a dynamic situation, as many stabbings are. Either the victim or his assailant might have been moving, or they could have been still and the knife itself moved in the wound. Sometimes the significance of such movement only emerges later, so it must be noted.

I detailed the two other stab wounds and their tracks: they had penetrated only the muscle of the back. Then I numbered the 'blunt' injuries to the left side of the face.

There were lacerations, abrasions and contusions on this body. There were stab wounds. But, notably, no defence wounds. Classic defence wounds are easy to spot – in a knife attack the palms and the fingers of the hand can be slashed as a victim attempts to grasp the blade of the knife in a desperate attempt at self-protection. This young man had no defence wounds, but then, the main attack had been from behind.

Now for my conclusions. That's the part of the report most people turn to first, the part laymen – police, and relatives, and so on – should be able to understand.

I knew the form by now. First exclude any chance that the victim died from a naturally occurring disease. Next, say what did actually cause death and how quickly the victim might have been expected to die. Then make any useful comment about possible weapons or events or actions that led to the injuries. Finally, give a medical opinion on the cause of death. This is the formal, legal, part of the report that will – if it is accepted – appear on the death certificate.

I wrote:

Death was not due to natural causes. Stab wound 1 . . . has caused haemorrhage. Death would have occurred in a matter of minutes. The appearance of the wounds is consistent with a weapon with a single cutting edge approximately 18 to 20mm in width at a distance of 15 to 17cm from the tip. The weapon must have been at least 15cm in length and most probably had a pointed tip.

Both the injuries to the right side and injuries (i) to (iv) on the left side of the face are consistent with a blow by or against a flat surface. The possibility that they were caused by collapse onto the roadway is unlikely but cannot be completely excluded. These injuries appear to have been caused some time prior to injury (v) on the left side of the face. This injury is consistent with contact with a rough surface.

Cause of death:

1a Haemorrhage

1b Stab wound to chest.

This crime, although no doubt decimating for the victim's family, was actually routine for a forensic pathologist. My report was not the longest or most detailed I have ever written. But I think it took me half the night.

Once the lad had been formally identified I was able to use his name, but apart from that certainty I experienced self-doubt over every fact as well as over my deductions. Was I surmising too much? How sure was I that those facial injuries weren't caused when he fell in the road? Should I give possible explanations for why the knife moved in the chest cavity? And did I sound confident enough? I didn't want, once the police had put a man in the dock, counsel for the defence saying, 'Tell me,

Dr Shepherd: how many stabbing post-mortems had you carried out entirely alone before this one? What! *None?*'

Even though I had only just started my career, I had already understood that court appearances could be a minefield. It was one thing to write your post-mortem report in the office and quite another to deliver it as an expert witness under fire in court. I'd heard many court-room stories from older colleagues and was both looking forward to and dreading my first appearance in the witness box at a Crown court.

The police were soon questioning a suspect in the Croydon stabbing, a man in his thirties who apparently was not previously known to the victim. The young man had gone to see him at some nearby lock-up garages to buy a cheap, probably stolen, car radio.

The police asked me to examine the suspect's version of events and we agreed that it would be best to do this back at the scene. And so, a couple of days later, accompanied by the same detective superintendent himself, as well as a detective inspector and a detective sergeant, I returned to Croydon.

We stood by a dingy row of garages. Paint peeled off their doors.

'The accused is saying somebody else stabbed the lad after he'd left this garage. That he must have been stabbed near to the place we found him,' said the super.

I said, 'There was no blood in the garage, so that could be true.'

They looked disappointed. It was not the last time in my career I would disappoint detectives.

'Well, we think the accused stabbed him right here. But then . . . there's no bloodstains outside the garages. Or in the road. Or anywhere but underneath the body.'

I felt important. I felt like Simpson. Closely followed by the high-ranking officers, I paced the route (a hundred paces) and timed it at the slow speed expected of a dying man who had been stabbed through the lung (fifty-three seconds) – not forgetting to move more and more slowly at the end to allow for his increasing breathlessness and dizziness.

I turned to the detectives.

'You may be right: he could have been stabbed at the garage and got to the road where he was found.'

They smiled.

I wrote:

In my opinion it is entirely possible for an individual with a wound such as Injury 1 to have travelled this distance on foot before collapsing.

The lack of bloodstains on the route may be explained by two factors. First, there would have been little external bleeding from an upright individual following Injury 1 until the level of blood within the chest reached the site of the wound in the skin. Second, the deceased was wearing clothing, in particular a thick jacket, which would have absorbed a significant quantity of blood.

I need not have worried about my court appearance. The first trial collapsed when the jury was discharged on a technicality before I could give evidence. By the time the case came to trial again I was a veteran of so many homicides that defence counsel had no idea this had been my very first case.

I gave my evidence and the cross-examination went smoothly enough.

It looked clear-cut to me. I had seen the evidence against the defendant and thought it was compelling. And three stab wounds including one deep penetration of the victim's lung from behind gave the tabloids a chance to use one of their favourite phrases: 'frenzied attack'. It was certainly used by the prosecution too, in an attempt to disgust the jury.

I was astonished, therefore, when the defendant was acquitted. Evidently the jury had not been convinced of his guilt beyond reasonable doubt. I worried for a while about what had gone wrong and whether, because this was my first case, I had somehow failed to present an effective report. Or had I struck the wrong note with the jury? I would never know.

It happened that a couple of years later I was reading the *Evening Standard* on the bus when I noticed a name which looked familiar in a court report. I read how a slim and attractive young man of about eighteen had been knifed by a stranger three times. One stab wound, into the left lung, had very nearly proved fatal. By some miracle the victim had survived to identify his assailant: in fact, he was able to reveal that the man had hung over him and suggested that, since he was dying, a suitable last act might be to have sex.

I remembered that very first case of mine. Same

defendant. Same crime. Different – but very similar-looking and very lucky – victim.

I knew about the defendant's earlier murder charge. The jury, of course, did not when they found him guilty of attempted murder.

# 9

My second case was another stabbing. At about nine o'clock one night I was called to an ordinary London red-brick, terraced house, distinguishable from all the other houses in the road only by the presence of the police outside.

Inside was an unexpectedly ornate interior. On the banisters, blood. I followed the trail upstairs and, just inside a bedroom door, feet nearest, naked in a huge puddle of blood, lay a grey-haired man, face down.

I pushed the door open. The dull, patterned wallpaper darkened the room and large, heavy, wooden furniture darkened it further. Although cluttered, everything was in its place. The alarm clock. The radio. The framed photos. The small TV on a mahogany chest of drawers facing the bed.

Here was the room of a man who led a well-ordered, working life. But that well-ordered life had been extinguished and the working man was lying awash with his own blood.

It was difficult to tread round him. His back was patterned with spatters and rivulets of blood. There was blood on the wall. The bed was half covered by a duvet but this did not hide the huge, deep bloodstains over the sheets. On the floor, by an electrical socket, almost floating in blood, was a long, wooden-handled kitchen knife.

I turned the body over with great care. I could see one

gaping knife wound in his chest. I thought there were probably more wounds, hidden by blood.

Then I took his temperature. Since he was already naked, this was easy. Taking a rectal temperature, especially if it involves removing clothes, can create forensic chaos so I had already learned that quite often it is better to get the body straight to the mortuary and take the temperature there. Now I saw that the victim's temperature was 26.6°C.

The detective who was watching me said, 'So, Doc, what time did he die, exactly?'

My heart sank. Especially at the word 'exactly'. That's the question everyone asks first. That's the question everyone thinks we can answer. That's the question which reveals the huge gap between the public perception of pathologists and the truth. I blame those TV cop shows. The fact is, it is very hard indeed for us to determine with any accuracy when a death occurred.

The detective was waiting.

I said, 'Well . . . I can't be sure . . .'

Body temperature may be the best forensic indicator we have for estimating the time of death but it is not a very reliable one. Basic physics tells us that a hot body will cool as its heat passes into the cooler environment. But of course, it's not that simple. A generalization would be that a body feels cold to touch within eight hours of death. It's not that simple, either. In fact, a body may not feel cold for as much as thirty-six hours and residual metabolic activity may mean the temperature never drops to the ambient level. Then, when decomposition is underway, the temperature will even start to rise.

There are so many variables that can affect the rate at which we cool after death: body temperature when death occurs, the environmental temperature, fluctuations in the weather, central heating, open windows, the amount of clothing on the body, the tog value of a duvet over it, the posture of the body (as we all instinctively know, a curled position retains more heat), bodyweight (fat is a good insulator), muscle bulk (less muscle means faster cooling) and the age of the deceased (children have a larger surface area to body weight and so lose heat more quickly) . . . a multitude of small factors make it a mug's game to estimate the time of death from the temperature of a body.

Even a computer program, after taking countless variables into account, would still not be able to give an accurate answer about the time of death. It may suggest that death occurred between a range of times but those times would probably be many hours apart. And still no one would expect accuracy of more than 90 per cent.

The detective nodded wisely. He said, 'I expect you'll be able to tell from the rigor mortis.'

Well, no. That's another misconception. Rigor mortis is one of death's most obvious processes but it is so highly variable that it is an even less reliable basis than body temperature for estimating the time of death. Its speed and onset are determined by temperature. A body outside in a cold winter may have no rigor after a week, although there can be a rapid onset of rigor as the body warms up when it is brought into the higher temperature of the mortuary. And there are other confounding factors. Was the deceased exercising just prior to death? Rigor mortis will be faster due to the lactic acid produced by physical exertion. Was death associated with a high fever? Again, rigor will be faster. Was electrocution the cause of death? This speeds up rigor, perhaps because of the stimulation of the muscle cells. Did death take place in front of a warm fire? Faster rigor. In a hot bath? Faster rigor.

Rigor mortis is actually caused by complex changes that occur once the heart has stopped beating and the muscle cells are deprived of the oxygen they need in order to metabolize. For years rigor was assumed to start in the face, as anyone making a delayed attempt at mouth-to-mouth resuscitation may recognize. We now understand that it develops uniformly throughout the body but that it is simply most detectable in the smaller muscles first – and these small muscles are found mainly in the jaw and around the eyes and fingers. As a generalization, rigor can be felt in these areas about three hours after death. It then appears to spread down the body from the head to the legs, although in fact this is just the differential stiffening of larger and larger muscle groups. The stiffening of the muscles generally occurs faster than the body cools, so there is usually a period when the body is both warm and stiff. And it doesn't last for ever: rigor mortis wears off after a day or so and the muscles become flaccid again.

In a temperate climate like the UK, rigor mortis may have affected all of the muscles – 'fully established' rigor – within twelve hours. In hot equatorial regions, rigor can be fully established and then disappear in just one hour. And it may sometimes seem that certain people – the very young, the very old or the emaciated – don't have it at all, because they have so little muscle bulk.

Its strength can be surprising: there are famous pictures of full rigor with the head on one chair and feet on another and the unsupported body in between as straight as a board. So, performing a post-mortem on a body in a state of rigor mortis poses its own problems – unless the deceased has obligingly died on his back with his arms by his sides.

The easiest choice is to wait for rigor to pass. Unfortunately, waiting is not an option for the forensic pathologist helping in a homicide investigation, where speed is of the essence.

That night I soon left the blood-filled bedroom for the mortuary. The deceased arrived very shortly after me. His neck, arms, jaw and knees had rigor mortis and he had actually died with one arm behind him and one folded in front. His right leg was raised.

I needed him to lie flat for the post-mortem and so I had to break rigor. This can require some strength. If an arm is bent I must push firmly on the joint until I break the chemical bonds between the molecules of actin and myosin in the cells. Once that bond is broken, the arm can be laid down flat on the table. But sometimes if the rigor is particularly strong – for instance, if the deceased is a muscled young man whose job involved heavy lifting – I'll need a mortuary assistant to help me. Breaking rigor involves putting considerable pressure on a specific joint to loosen the muscle and it then gives way gradually, not suddenly like a bone snapping.

In this case the patient was sixty-two years old and rigor was quite easily broken by vigorously moving the arms backwards and forwards until they felt loose.

At the repeated request of the police officers, I used the two unreliable guides – body temperature and stiffness – to arrive at a range of times between which death might have occurred. Bearing in mind that there are any number of variables, of course. In this case, I gave an estimated time since death of four to six hours.

'Well done, Doc,' said the senior detective, who was just coming into the post-mortem room after taking a phone call. 'The bloke who killed him says it was about four thirty, five o'clock this afternoon.'

'You've got him already?'

'He's just turned himself in. They were in a homosexual relationship. Says he lost his temper.'

It was quite a serious loss of temper. There were eight stab wounds, one of them a really gaping wound on the outside which inside had directly penetrated the heart. So clearly do knives leave their tracks and hilts their bruises that I was able to sketch with detailed dimensions the weapon which had been used by the murderer. It was my first knife sketch ever based on wound tracks and I was amazed when it exactly matched the dimensions of the kitchen knife the police found at the scene. From now on, Shepherd was a knife man.

In addition, although this does seem to me, looking back, like ludicrous overenthusiasm, I thought I could establish exactly what had happened from the wounds themselves and from the blood staining around the room. That was, after all, what Professor Simpson would have done.

A tell-tale spattering on the wall said that the first and fatal injury was inflicted here. The wound was in the left upper chest and its track was slightly left to right. Classic. This told me that the killer was right-handed, that both he and the victim had been standing and that he had used an overarm downward thrust.

The victim then collapsed onto the left side of the bed. That was clear from the position of the bloodstains on the sheets. And from the thin lines of blood spattered on the ceiling above – 'cast-off staining', which is the result of blood flying from the blade's tip as the assailant raises the knife to stab again – it was easy to deduce that the killer had stood over his victim while stabbing him three more times.

The victim had rolled out of bed and crawled for the door. This was evidenced from the trail of blood he had left. The final four stab wounds were almost certainly inflicted here, by the door, where the victim had died in a pool of blood. But the killer might have saved himself the effort: the first thrust was fatal and after it penetrated his heart the victim had only minutes to live. The proximity and uniformity of these four wounds, all at the same angle, each a copy of the last, indicated that the victim was motionless by this point and perhaps already dead. And what about the blood I had seen smeared on the banisters? That had certainly been left by the bloodied departing boyfriend: it was all over for the victim before he had reached the door.

The killer had already confessed but, nevertheless, I was so proud of my deductions that after the post-mortem I insisted on telling the detective.

'Uh huh,' he said, without interest.

'Look, you can see here . . .' I held out the helpful diagram I had drawn. He did not take it.

Ever eager, I now offered to write a statement explaining my reconstruction of events.

He blinked and looked away.

'Nah, don't bother, Doc. No one will read it, the bloke's coughed.'

I was greatly disappointed. It was my first inkling that the police really do not want me to play Sherlock Holmes. Or even Keith Simpson. My hero was an invaluable part of the crime-solving team in the first half of the twentieth century and was involved throughout homicide investigations at every level: throwing theories around with high-ranking officers or counsel, discussing clues with detectives at the scene. I'd like to do that too. Sometimes I am bursting to tell the police exactly what my skills and training suggest happened. But police investigation has changed. The 'science' of homicide has now become such a specialized business that the many disciplines involved offer their separate facts and the police co-ordinate everyone's findings and come to their own conclusions. That can work – as long as the officers are skilled and experienced.

Next, the decision to charge or not is made by Crown Prosecution Service lawyers. Fine. As long as the lawyers don't struggle when confronted by complex medical issues.

I think the system would be most effective if we could all sit down together when a case is difficult and complicated – the police and the CPS with the pathologist, the forensic scientists, the blood-spatter specialist, the toxicologist, the ballistics expert – and discuss our facts together. But we seldom do that any longer.

# IO

Gradually, crime scenes and post-mortems became my working life. I was allocated easy cases to start with. They were all different but they were all straightforward. Routine, in fact. Except that there is really nothing routine about any crime scene, it's just how we all try to make it seem. A motionless body, sometimes hideously mutilated, lies at the centre of a web of bustling, serious professionals who are all engaging fully with it while somehow remaining detached from its horror.

And at the edges of this web, at a safe distance, is the grief and shock of the bereaved. Pathologists know that even the most routine cases carry a payload of trauma for someone. At that stage, I was still determined to stay uninvolved in this trauma if I could. I did know, however, that sooner or later there would have to be an interface with the living.

At home, there were growing children and a busy wife. I was a hands-on father, unusual perhaps then, but I had been brought up by a hands-on father myself and the result was that making time for my children was a bigger priority for me than for many others of my generation.

However, I did have to learn how to leave the mortuary behind me at home. I had to forget the sights and smells of the place, forget the homicide victim I had just been examining and whip off the mask of clinical detachment just as I walked in through the front door to the quotidian world of daylight and children. Of course, that wasn't easy. My mask was securely fixed. And so probably I didn't always remove it successfully. Certainly, my wife did have a problem with that. Jen understood why I had to be detached. But she told me scientific detachment was an approach I adopted far too often. At home. In our marriage. Which was now under strain.

A few years earlier, Jen, who had loved being a nurse and a health visitor, had shyly told me that she had always secretly wanted to be a doctor. She hadn't progressed well at school because her father held extremely conservative, indeed colonial, views on the 'right' sort of jobs for women and the education they required. She was also mildly dyslexic, which had further affected her early educational attainment.

I had no doubts about her abilities or her intelligence, and when she told me her ambition I promised to support her through the long years of hard slog ahead. Now, I was very proud of how she had worked her way through the Open University into a place at my alma mater, University College London. She was already on her way to qualifying as a doctor.

But, of course, this put us under great pressure: of time, of money. I earned a fair salary but nannies were expensive and, although Jen would be earning one day, she wasn't yet. Quite often my work clashed with her training and then one of us had to give way. Our lives were hectic and complicated and our relationship sagged beneath our loads. A forensic examination of our marriage would reveal clusters of quick discussions, one of us always rushing in as the other rushed out, communication often limited to little more than times, dates, parents' meetings, school sports days, logistics. Clinical interaction of that sort.

A beautiful summer's Sunday morning. The children, still small, streaking into the garden like arrows as soon as I opened the back door. Me, a fresh-faced pathologist, always at the ready to rush to a crime scene and getting a whoosh of adrenalin if the phone rang when I was on call. Jen, almost a doctor, always studying.

I was just about to make breakfast.

Outside, the children cried, 'Oh no!'

The phone was ringing. At this time of the morning. It could only mean one thing.

I considered the possibilities. Probably, because it was Sunday, someone had simply died after a Saturday-night fight. Upstairs, I knew Jen must be sighing. I imagined her sitting with her elbows on the desk, her head sinking into her hands.

I did feel bad. She had been up since the crack of dawn with her books and I had promised to look after the children today. If the phone didn't ring. But it had, and now Jen was about to take the shrapnel from a drunken brawl.

A voice told me that the victim was a young Caucasian male. So, there had almost certainly been a pub-brawl last night. Except for one thing. The caller had identified himself as a detective chief inspector. A detective chief inspector who said, as the call ended, that he would be waiting for me at the mortuary with a detective chief superintendent. Top brass. At the weekend. There must be something unusual about this case.

'Which mortuary?' asked Jen, getting up from her books. 'Westminster?'

'Swindon.'

She did a double take.

'*Swindon*? In *Wiltshire*?'

I nodded.

She sighed. 'See you this evening, then.'

When I arrived in Swindon, the two senior detectives were waiting, along with a police officer and the coroner's officer. The mortuary staff handed me a cup of tea and the chief superintendent began.

'Young man. Over the drink-drive limit, took a corner on a country lane badly. His girlfriend was in the front seat and basically . . . well, have you got her statement, John?'

The detective inspector nodded and opened a file. He shuffled through some pages of typing.

'So . . . the lad was working all night on Friday and he's probably been up all day on Saturday and he's had a few drinks so now he's tired and drunk and it's six o'clock. Good light but the road's a bit damp. He's picked up the girl and he's taking her back to his place for a cosy Saturday night. They're going round a bend and the van's coming towards them and she says . . .'

His finger found its way down the page.

'"I shouted, 'Oh my God, Michael, look out!' and he immediately jerked the car to the left. Michael's side of the car hit the driver's side of the van. At the time of the impact I closed my eyes. When I opened them, both vehicles were at a standstill, although there was still glass flying around inside the car. I looked at Michael and his head was back and his eyes were closed. I thought he was unconscious. I shook him and he sat bolt upright as if I had just woken him up."

'"I saw the other driver get out. And then this man appeared. I don't know where he came from. He was wearing trousers with no shirt and he was really brown, he gave the appearance of being a labourer."'

The chief superintendent said, 'He was actually working in his garden nearby and heard the crash.'

His colleague nodded and read on.

'"This man asked if I was all right. Michael got out through the window and walked to the front of the car. He pulled bits off it and kicked it and seemed to be very angry and upset. I was upset too. I was hysterical. Michael was kicking and throwing a paddy."

'"I got out and lit a cigarette and gave one to Michael and then this man with no shirt said, 'Don't light your cigarettes, there's petrol at the back of the car here.'"'

'"Michael told him to mind his own business and the man with no shirt said something to Michael, I didn't hear what, which aggravated him and then a fight started."'

The detective stopped reading and looked at me. They both looked at me as if they expected me to say something.

'What actually happened in this fight?' I asked.

'Michael tried to hit the man with no shirt and missed. The man hit him back, that's all.'

That can't have been all. Why were they reluctant to tell me more? I asked, 'Well, what does the girlfriend say?'

The detective read, '"The man with no shirt clenched his right fist and hit Michael full in the face, either on his nose or his mouth. Another man, with streaked hair, had pulled up in his car by now and he got behind Michael and put his arms right round Michael to hold him and Michael went a funny colour, a purply red, and passed out. The man let him sort of fall to the floor."'

The detective stopped reading again. But I knew there was more.

'Any further description?' I prompted.

'"By this time, it was raining heavily. The man with no shirt started shaking Michael quite violently to try and get some response from him. He was saying, 'Come on, get up!' but Michael didn't move and I could see he was really hurt, he looked really poorly. The reddish purple tinge had faded. They couldn't revive him. An old man in a Sierra stopped and put his jacket on him to keep him warm until the ambulances came. When my ambulance drove away, Michael's ambulance was still there."'

The chief superintendent took up the story: 'Never recovered consciousness. Swindon sent him to Oxford for a CT scan, then he came back to Swindon. He died here this morning.'

He handed me some medical notes from Oxford. I looked at them and nodded.

'So you want to know whether you've got a road traffic accident on your hands or a homicide?'

I saw them flinch at the word homicide. I wondered again why we had the top brass here. Was the deceased famous? Especially well connected?

The superintendent said, 'The girlfriend's making a right fuss, saying the bloke with no shirt killed Michael and now the family's making a big fuss too.'

I got up. 'Well, let's take a look at him.'

'Right,' said PC Masters as we walked into the room where the young man's body lay waiting for us. 'This is Michael Ross.'

I did not recognize the name but I half expected to recognize the face. There were cuts and bruises but I could still see that the young man had handsome rock-star looks, with thick dark hair curling around his forehead. However, there was nothing familiar about him.

'How old is he?'

'He's twenty-four.'

I began to scribble and, when I looked up, saw that the photographer had arrived and was waiting for me to tell him what pictures I wanted.

'Whole body front. Then we'll do close-ups of the face and the neck and we'll have those bruises on his knees, please. Oh, and this fight he got into . . .'

'The alleged fight,' said the detective chief superintendent quickly.

'. . . please photograph the hands so that we can see his knuckles.'

I scribbled:

Recent superficial abrasions, mostly vertical over the forehead, bridge of the nose and left side of the chin. Recent punctate area of bruising (8 x 2cm) lying diagonally over the right lower neck.

I marked Michael's wounds on my blank body outlines then looked closely at his teeth.

'No sign that he was hit in the mouth,' I said. The room

seemed to rustle a bit but when I looked up everyone was still.

There were a number of other old bruises and scars on the body, which I noted, as well as details of Michael's tattoos. His back seemed unmarked. We photographed this and I then turned him over again and began the post-mortem. The officers watched with stony faces. There is usually at least one who turns green and this time, surprisingly, it was the super.

'I'll have to get used to it all over again; I haven't been to one of these for years,' he said apologetically. 'I've just come back from the fraud squad.'

Ever since the young PC had thrown up in the first forensic post-mortem I carried out alone, I had given a lot of thought to post-mortem revulsion, a condition which can affect anyone whose job requires them to be present.

I asked myself why I had never, not once, shared their revulsion. Answer: because I was so fascinated by the workings of the human body in general and my findings in particular. I decided that if I could somehow share this fascination with others in the room, I might be able to help them past their horror. My theory was that, if I could involve them in the proceedings through knowledge and understanding, then they would no longer be helpless, shocked onlookers.

The nervous silence in which I conducted my first post-mortem and the nausea of the PC who witnessed it could not have been sheer coincidence. So I had determined that the next time someone present became really upset, I'd put my plan into action by talking. Politely but lamely muttering, 'Er . . . are you all right?' as the super's cheeks took on a greenish tinge would not do.

Adopting what I hoped was a reassuring tone, I said, 'As some of you will know, I have to check the organs inside the body – not just for injuries from the car crash, not just for damage from the subsequent brawl, but to ascertain that there wasn't some other, less obvious, contributing factor to this death – like a natural disease. So, I'll be taking a good look at all his organs.'

The super nodded. Rather slowly. The room was silent, as though a blanket had been thrown over it.

'Got any music?' I asked the mortuary staff. 'Something classical would be nice.'

They switched on Radio 1. I glanced at the super. Maybe the sound of inane voices would steady his nerves. I did ask them to turn it down a bit, though.

Cutting dead skin is like cutting the skin on a chicken joint: easy if you use a sharp knife. The cut is hampered, if at all, not by its strength but by the skin's natural elasticity, and as a healthy young man Michael Ross's skin did have that elasticity. As I sliced through the fat which lies beneath – in all of us to some extent, even someone as slim as Michael – I glanced up. The super was not doing too well. Radio 1 wasn't helping. It was time to start talking again to test my theory that information, any information, is soothing.

'I'm nearly into the chest cavity now. From this stage, without impinging on Michael's dignity at all, you could try to forget that we are dissecting a human. You've cut meat often enough and this is no different in colour or consistency. You'll soon see that the liver is like any liver you buy in Sainsbury's. The kidneys too. And this muscle I'm cutting now, well I always think it's a bit like a good steak.'

'Chips, anyone?' said the detective inspector jovially.

No one replied but the superintendent tried to nod again. As if we were making polite conversation. However, he could not pursue this convention by meeting my eye because his own eyes were now fixed on Michael Ross.

I continued my work. PC Masters was keen to ignore the boss's discomfort but the coroner's officer seemed to take a certain amount of pleasure in it.

'It's all right, he can't feel a thing,' he told the super cheerfully. 'Bloody good anaesthetic, death.'

I glanced at the super. Hmm. Start talking.

'Of course, I'll have to look closely at Michael's brain and his neck. According to the medical notes, that's where I should expect to find damage caused by the road traffic accident and by the fight. I mean, alleged fight. But I can only be guided by the notes, not bound by them. I still have to examine every organ carefully in case the doctors missed something.'

No one in the room, not even the coroner's officer, looked as though the prospect of examining Michael's brain was very attractive. I decided not to even try telling them how fascinating this would be.

Michael had been a healthy enough lad although, despite his young age, a hard-drinking lifestyle was already having its effect. His heart was slightly enlarged and his liver fatty, both probably signs of significant alcohol consumption. I was sure the brain would prove the most interesting organ and, as expected, when I lifted it out

I found that it was full of blood. The door slammed. I didn't even have to turn round to know who had left the room.

I asked the photographer for a picture of the brain whole, knowing that I would have to section it soon to study its histology. I'd probably get a colleague who was an expert in brain pathology to take a look at the slides too. I also needed to carry out a really detailed examination of Michael's neck, far too detailed for this post-mortem. So I prepared a fixative in order to transport it. The remaining police officers drew back at the intense smell of the formalin as I turned the body over and carefully removed the neck structures with the accompanying arteries, placing this in a mortuary bucket to make sure I disturbed the vertebrae as little as possible.

'Glad I drove here, I can put this in the boot,' I said, as the mortuary assistant carried the bucket away to seal it.

'You never would have taken it on the train!' exclaimed PC Masters.

'I sometimes have to,' I admitted. 'It looks a bit strange but I just hope the other passengers assume I've been out catching tadpoles in the country.' Certainly, no one would ever guess what's in the bucket. Unless they could smell it.

'Right then,' said the cheerful mortuary assistant. 'Cups of tea all round.'

I went into the locker room to change and wash. The police officers had appropriated the mortuary's bereavement room since it was empty, and I found them here sitting in a circle drinking their tea. It was a quiet room, decorated in dull shades. Along one wall was a large tank, two fish swimming up and down it noiselessly. I don't know why there is nearly always a fish tank in bereavement rooms.

The chief superintendent's cheeks were deathly pale. He was not so much sitting in his seat as propped up by it and he was evidently disinclined to speak, glancing at the detective inspector instead.

The detective inspector asked, 'So, what do you think, Doc?'

'It will take a while to get you my full report because I've a lot of work to do on the brain and the neck to confirm my findings. But I can give you an informal, off-the-record debrief if you like.'

'Yes please,' he said quickly, exchanging glances with the super. What was it about this case that was causing the top brass so much concern?

'Well, I don't believe that the punch-up – alleged punch-up – had anything to do with Michael Ross's death. He was killed by the impact of the car accident,' I said.

The detective inspector tried to stop himself but he couldn't. He smiled. Even the super, still pale and barely sipping his tea, managed to pull his mouth into an approximation of a grin.

'Are you sure?' the inspector asked happily. 'How can you be sure?'

'You can see just by looking at him that Michael screeched to a halt very suddenly – he's got a seat belt injury on the right side of his neck to prove it. I believe that the sudden stop caused severe whiplash to the spine. Once his spine was out of alignment – and according to his girlfriend he was turning the wheel frantically at the time, which might have given his spine an additional rotational problem – the arteries, or at least one of them, running up the sides of the vertebrae, were ruptured. A ruptured artery bleeds into a space around the brain: he had a sub-arachnoid haemorrhage and that is what killed him.'

'Whiplash. It was whiplash!' said the inspector, beaming at the super.

'A brain haemorrhage . . .' muttered the super weakly.

'Caused by impact!' the detective finished for him.

I said, 'You can get a sub-arachnoid haemorrhage for genetic reasons and I can't 100 per cent rule out a congenital problem yet. But it's also caused by trauma and in this case the haemorrhage was almost certainly a result of the accident.'

PC Masters was looking more serious than his bosses. He had been watching the fish swim up and down their tank.

'Doc . . . how do you know the haemorrhage wasn't caused by a trauma in the fight; I mean, alleged fight?'

'If the fight had caused the haemorrhage then there would have been a lot more soft tissue injury. There's just one bruise on the face, which might have been a blow from a fist. I think it's too minor to have done much but I'll be checking carefully when I examine the neck. Virtually all the other facial injuries look like windscreen glass to me.'

The inspector said, 'But Michael Ross's family's asking how he was able to climb out of the car, walk about, smoke, talk, argue, fight. If he had a brain haemorrhage. Until the other bloke, the one with no shirt, hit him.'

'A delayed death is fairly classic for this type of haemorrhage. It can take a few minutes, or even hours sometimes, for blood to spread from the damaged artery up the canal to the skull. He managed to do all those things during the lucidity period that sometimes precedes death from a sub-arachnoid haemorrhage.'

They all looked at one another.

'So . . . you're sure it's nothing to do with the fight?'

'I don't think so. But these haemorrhages are found after both pub brawls and road traffic accidents, so I'll have to do a lot more tests before I can be sure I'm right. I believe the tests will show that Michael was a dying man from the moment of the accident and the fight made no difference.'

That's what I thought. The timing, however, was unfortunate, since he seemed to die at the moment the man hit him. I was going to have to work hard to prove my theory, and be prepared to change it, since there was sure to be a second post-mortem.

The policemen sat back in their chairs and looked at each other.

'If you had manslaughter charges lined up against the man with no shirt, I'd drop them now because they probably won't stand up. I suppose you might get him for assault,' I offered.

They said nothing.

I asked, 'Michael Ross had the looks and liver of a rock star: is he famous?'

They shook their heads.

'So . . . why do we have a chief superintendent and chief inspector here on a Sunday morning?'

The super looked at me. So did the inspector. Who paused, then said, 'Off the record, Doc, we're here because I thought we were in a spot of bother.'

I waited. The officers looked uncomfortable. Finally, the super spoke.

'The man with no shirt. The one who hit Michael. He was an off-duty police officer.'

So that was it.

'We didn't tell you before because we didn't want to influence you.'

I said stiffly, 'You wouldn't have influenced me. Pathology tells its own story.' No, that sounded all wrong. Far too pompous, far too much like someone who was occasionally unnerved by the number of versions of the truth he was beginning to encounter. I added, 'Even if I wanted to ignore inconvenient truths, there's usually a second post-mortem, so I couldn't do that.'

But the super was not listening. His face still deathly white and his voice low, he said, 'You don't know how worried I've been about this one. It would look so bad for the force and, between ourselves, a few things have been said about that officer in the past; he loses his rag and . . . of course, we didn't want to believe he'd killed a man but his record isn't . . . well anyway, what you've told us is a big relief, Doc.'

'The thing is,' said the police constable, who clearly knew the man with no shirt, 'I can see how it happened. The driver, Michael Ross, he was an idiot to smoke near the car when there was fuel all over the road, and when Mitch told him that, he tried to argue. So Mitch had to make him stop. I can see that.'

'Persuading an RTA victim to behave safely is one thing, losing your rag with him is another,' said the inspector.

Now they knew the officer's action had not contributed to the death, they seemed able to discuss the matter. Even the super joined in a little.

'Are you going to be all right?' I asked him as I left.

He nodded but I thought his face still looked pale and drawn. I wondered then if attending a post-mortem could actually be a traumatizing experience. I had to ensure somehow that it wasn't. I had done my best today. How could I do more?

I heard the officers' voices still debating as I walked down the corridor. I drove home with my bucket and its strange cargo in the boot.

'Pooh, Daddy, you're really smelly,' said my daughter. Anna's never been one to mince words. Jen fell gratefully on her books and I made supper and then, when I was no longer on call, allowed the children to persuade me that we should take the dog to the park.

I loaded all three into the car.

'Anna, seat belt,' I said.

'No.'

'Seat belt.'

'Don't like my seat belt.'

'It's not the law to wear a belt,' piped up Chris. 'Because we're in the back seat.' Which in those days was true.

'It's the law,' I said firmly, 'in this car. Seat belts! Now! Or we don't move.'

Michael Ross was not saved by his seat belt but I had already seen many, many fatalities that could have been prevented by wearing one. Travelling without a seat belt is a risk I would never take.

'I'm not going to put my seat belt on!' Anna declared. 'Anyway, it's not fair, because Dilly doesn't have to wear a seat belt.'

Dilly wagged her tail.

I said, 'Right. Then we don't move.' And to show how ready and willing I was to sit in the car until she was safely buckled in, I got out my cigarettes, lit one, and proceeded to puff on it until my daughter had fully complied with my health-and-safety rules. Then we drove to the park. I know, I know. But at least I opened the windows.

From this you will see that my attitude to risk-taking – my own and my children's – has always been as idiosyncratic as everyone else's. At least working with death has helped me recognize it can arrive most unexpectedly and therefore I do appreciate the good things life has to offer. So that evening I enjoyed the park, I enjoyed the general laughter while bathing the children and I enjoyed reading them stories and then kissing them goodnight as they snuggled into bed.

Later, Jen took a break and we sat together in the garden. As usual on a Sunday, we were synchronizing diaries, working out how we were going to manage our various commitments. We couldn't afford after-hours childcare, so each week our time had to be planned and managed.

When we had finished, we sat back. With our cigarettes. The evening was so still that the smoke rose upwards in a straight line. It was good to relax as the sun went down. And it was inconceivable to us that it might be possible to relax without cigarettes. We were fully aware of the effect of this: I often found myself looking at lungs which bore the strangely beautiful but deadly patina of smoke inhalation.

But we regarded cigarettes as an essential part of our full and busy lives.

The next day I did some research into sub-arachnoid haemorrhages. I found that victims often show aggression in that period when they appear to be recovering, the period between accident and death during which Michael Ross had started fighting. And alcohol, which frequently plays a role in these haemorrhages, can certainly make matters worse by increasing blood pressure and making rupture of any damaged area more likely.

It seemed Michael was a textbook case but I still had a lot of work to do. I not only had to X-ray the whiplash injury to the spine but I had to take a series of cross-sections of the spine's arteries to find the resulting rupture and show how it had caused the haemorrhage.

The chief superintendent phoned me.

'Michael Ross's family wants another post-mortem. They think we're closing ranks and they say that if we don't charge the off-duty police officer with manslaughter, they'll file a civil case against him.'

'Did you explain that I found –'

'They weren't interested in hearing anything from me. They've got their own pathologist.'

'That's not unusual.'

He named the pathologist the family was consulting.

I was pleased. 'Oh, I know him and he's very good.'

The super sounded less pleased. 'Wants to do his post-mortem the day after tomorrow.'

'I'll be there.'

When there is a second post-mortem – and there often is, for example lawyers defending clients on a murder charge frequently call for one – it is normal but not required for the first pathologist to be present. I thought it would be both useful and interesting to watch a post-mortem performed by this esteemed colleague.

Before the second post-mortem, I examined the brain further, reassuring myself that there was no congenital aneurysm that had caused the haemorrhage. And I continued with my slow and careful dissection of the vertebral arteries, photographing every step of the way, until I found the rupture which had caused the haemorrhage. I sent specimens and photos to the Ross family's forensic pathologist and to another neuropathological expert who was also coming to the second post-mortem.

Afterwards, the expert and the family's pathologist conferred and then wrote a detailed report that confirmed all my results. The pathologist agreed that whiplash, caused not just by Michael's sudden braking but his frantic turning of the steering wheel, had dislocated his spine. This dislocation ruptured an artery carrying blood to the brain, resulting in a haemorrhage.

He said, 'The walking about, smoking, talking, arguing and fighting may have accelerated the rate of haemorrhage but I doubt very much whether the fatal outcome could have been avoided. After a few minutes, the amount of haemorrhage became such that Mr Ross lost consciousness and from then on the fatal outcome was inevitable.'

My post-mortem had pleased the police and the cause of death was certainly beyond dispute when the second post-mortem concurred. But supposing the forensic evidence had not been so clear-cut and the police had put pressure on me to exonerate their officer? A slight adjustment in wording at the end of a report ('There is a possibility that . . .' to 'It is unlikely that . . .') can be enough for the Crown Prosecution Service to bring charges or to drop them. How hard would it have been to resist such pressure if it came from the Met, fostered by the hopes and fears of individuals I worked with on a regular and friendly basis?

I reminded myself that I became a forensic pathologist to be a seeker of the truth. That meant I must stand up for the truth whatever pressure I was placed under to massage it. I see now that this is just the sort of noble thought a keen young man of limited experience might have. I had not worked on enough cases to know how malleable a concept truth is for some people, nor how open to interpretation, instinct and inclination are all truths, even those that appear to be scientific fact. Although there had already been some intimations of truth's elasticity. In court, for instance. But overall I was still deluding myself that it was always possible to find a moral pathway that everyone would recognize as clear and correct.

# II

Someone had to go and speak to a CID training course, and I was pleased it was my turn. There are a lot of police courses and officers have no choice about attending – but some make it obvious they would rather be playing golf or even out on the job than sitting in a lecture hall.

I was sure of getting their attention today, however, because my subject was the human body after death. The police are seldom present when someone dies. They inevitably arrive after the event, sometimes a long time afterwards. This lecture was designed to help them recognize what they might find.

I began by explaining that death is a process. And when that process, dying, is complete, it sets off another series of processes which eventually return us to the earth and complete the life cycle.

The screen lit up above me and the police officers stretched out their legs. A few sipped their coffee and relaxed with the air of men settling down with their wives to watch a David Attenborough wildlife documentary.

I didn't want to give them too much science, so I simply said that oxygen is vital for almost all cells. It facilitates the cells' multitude of life-sustaining chemical reactions: this is metabolism. On death, when there is no oxygen, muscle cells rapidly become flaccid. They may, for some hours, still respond. To touch. Or the discharge of a dying motor neurone cell. Or other forms of stimulation. As a result, disconcertingly, limbs may even twitch in a lifeless body.

The eyelids may close or, more often, half-close, because muscles in the eyelid are too flaccid to complete the movement. The response to light is lost; however, there is a myth in some cultures, predominately Asian but also in the West, that the eyes retain the final image they see, so exposing the face of their killer. This was considered as a scientific possibility in Europe in the 1870s. It was called Optography and experiments were performed on individuals before and after execution, but without success. Despite the lack of any scientific proof, the concept took root in the public imagination, thanks in part to authors such as Rudyard Kipling and Jules Verne, who used it in short stories. The idea even featured in an episode of *Doctor Who* in the 1970s. Once cemented in the public psyche, it has been very difficult to remove. Another old wives' tale is that hair continues to grow after death. In fact, the cells in hair follicles die with the rest of the skin. The skin, if the deceased is Caucasian, becomes pale on death because blood is not circulating and blood pressure is lost.

The rings of muscle that control the passage of food and liquid through the digestive system lose their tone, which means that, depending on both the angle of the body and the individual's internal organs, urine may leak out. Faeces also, but this is less common because of the structure of the rectum.

Another common leak is that of semen. So, it is never safe for the pathologist to assume, on finding semen outside the body, that the deceased had sex just before he died – although he might have done. And, just because gastric contents are found in the mouth, there can be no assumption that vomiting was a cause of death, since regurgitation is found in about 25 per cent of post-mortems.

The police officers really did not need reminding that death can be a messy business. They knew that bodies often leak from orifices in a way their owners would find shameful in life. In fact, I long ago understood, after talking to people about their end-of-life fears, that this undignified leakage is something many find worrying about death. But I believe there is no need for anxiety. Those of us who choose to work with the dead are non-judgemental and respectful and I feel that worriers really won't care about this when life is actually draining away from them. I think they will be entirely involved in the process of letting go and giving up their bodies. Embarrassment is just the kind of worldly concern which I believe the dying relinquish, often perhaps with relief.

The next process after death is cooling. I could have devoted an entire lecture to this subject but I offered only the most general of guidelines: I wanted the police officers to recognize how unrealistic TV movies are about judging the time of death accurately from a body's temperature. The next process is the stiffening of the muscles known as rigor mortis: they were familiar with that one. Then I showed pictures of hypostasis.

On death, blood stops circulating and its components, cells and protein, become subject to the normal laws of gravity. Which means that the red blood cells sink and settle in the lowest areas of the body. The tiny blood vessels in the skin in those areas then become distended by blood. This makes the skin initially appear pink but within five or six hours it turns a very angry colour, bright pink with a bluish tinge. And here is the paint box we call hypostasis.

Its alarming appearance is heightened, in Caucasians, by the great whiteness of adjacent parts of the body, those which are pressed against a firm surface – a bed or the floor perhaps – where the blood vessels are squashed flat and so cannot fill. These areas stay blanched. A Caucasian who dies lying in bed therefore has hypostasis staining most of the skin on the back, as well as the back of the neck, thighs and lower legs – and very white skin on the buttocks as well as white patches over the shoulders. In darker-skinned people, hypostasis is, of course, still present, but its appearance is much less livid.

Hypostasis does eventually disappear. But only when the blood is dispersed by the final process after death. This process is decomposition. Many people find the idea of decomposition repellent. It might help to remember that this is an important natural process that completes the life cycle of the human body and returns it to the chemical pool that is the earth. It is hard to imagine what our world would be like without the ultimately cleansing process of decomposition, smelly and ugly though it may seem to the living.

There are three ways a body can decompose: by putrefaction, mummification or adipocere, of which putrefaction is by far the most common.

I had brought pictures and the officers seemed unaffected by those I had shown so far. But I watched them sit up now, hoping, I guessed, they wouldn't have to look at putrefaction. But a putrefying body is simply one in which the soft tissues are turning slowly to liquid. The speed of this process of course depends on temperature. In the UK, bodies will usually start to putrefy around three or four days after death and this will be visible to the naked eye quickly. I showed a picture of a body and, with the pointer, drew the officers' attention to one small area of green discolouration just on the right side of the lower abdomen.

'It's usually just there,' I said. 'That's where you'll first see putrefaction.'

Our guts are full of bacteria, which are vital for digestion. Now, in death, those bacteria break out of the bowel and into the abdominal cavity and then the blood vessels. The process starts at this certain point on the abdomen, near the appendix, because the abdominal wall is very close to the intestine here. Putrefaction can begin elsewhere, but only with good reason: for example, if a body is lying across a heating pipe, or part of it is in direct sunlight. Wherever it begins, by the time the green blotch is visible on the skin, then the bacteria are running riot inside the body.

The blood vessels provide easy channels for the bacteria to spread, causing the haemoglobin there to decompose. Visible result: the extraordinary and beautiful fern-like pattern of the veins closest to the surface becomes clearly etched on the skin as though tattooed in brown. It is often evident on the arms and thighs.

I think the police officers were beginning to realize now that this was no David Attenborough documentary. But, like every death process, this rather beautiful stage is temporary. Gradually the pattern is lost as the skin blisters into red and brown fluid. As the blisters burst, the skin sloughs off.

One waste product of all this bacterial activity is gas, and so now the body begins to swell. First the genitals become bloated, followed by the face, abdomen and breasts. Then eyes and tongue protrude as bloody liquid is forced up from the lungs, leaking from nose and mouth. The face, with its popping eyes and tongue, has a look of amazement.

Those officers who could look at the screen – and many chose not to – stared back at the body I showed them with equal amazement. Swelling bodies at this stage of decomposition become so dark that anyone finding one can wrongly assume a skinny Caucasian was in life an overweight black man.

Flies have a role to play in putrefaction by feasting and laying their eggs, which turn into maggots with voracious appetites. Animals, domestic and wild, may also make an important contribution to bodily breakdown (outside there are rats and foxes and inside . . . well, yes, a starving dog which finds itself locked in the house after a death will probably eat its owner to survive).

Within about a week of death – depending as usual on the weather and micro-environment – body cavities will burst and tissues will start to liquefy. Within about a month, the soft tissues are all liquid and these will drain off into the ground. The usual order of decomposition is first the intestines, stomach, liver, blood and heart. Then the lungs and air passages. Next the brain, then the kidneys and bladder. Finally the muscles. The prostate, the uterus, the tendons and the ligaments are relatively resistant to putrefaction and may not break down for months to leave the skeleton stripped. I didn't show any pictures of this final part of the process. They looked as though they had seen enough.

A much more unusual form of decomposition in this country is mummification. Mummified bodies are brown and dry. The skin is drawn tightly over the skeleton so it looks shrivelled and tough like leather. This process dries the tissues, hardening them in a way that prevents putrefaction. It usually requires hot, desert-like conditions: bodies buried in the sands of Egypt may even mummify spontaneously.

In the UK, mummification can happen if a thin person (the thin are more likely to cool and desiccate quickly) dies in a very dry and draughty place – an attic or chimney, for instance. It is rare to find a mummified body now but not so long ago they were encountered relatively often.

'Anyone here seen a mummified body outside the British Museum?' I asked my audience. A few raised their hands.

One of the older officers said, 'Baby. Been hidden in the attic. And not yesterday, either. Years and years ago, probably during the war they said, because it happened a lot then.'

'Was it a newborn?' I asked.

He nodded. I had actually recently seen a mummified newborn myself, and the circumstances had been the same. The bodies of newborn babies are relatively sterile, which makes them less susceptible to putrefaction and more likely to mummify. Those babies were generally born in secret to single mothers in the days when this was truly shameful. Either they were born dead, or they died at birth as the mother struggled to cope alone, or they were actually killed but, in many cases, burial was apparently not an option and so the body would be hidden under the floorboards or in the attic. As social attitudes to birth outside marriage changed, these discoveries decreased, but in the 1980s they still sometimes happened when old ladies died and young couples bought their houses for renovation – to find, in the loft, the tragic, long-hidden, mummified corpse of a tiny baby.

There are a few examples of adult homicides revealed years later by the discovery of a mummified body. Most famous is a case in Wales where a strangled woman was hidden in a cupboard for years while her family continued to claim her pension. Once completely dried, a mummified body can last a long time. But eventually mould forms and the dried tissues gradually become powdery and disintegrate. The mummy very often attracts rodents, beetles and moths, too. However, if it is recovered in time it can very faithfully reveal through preserved bruises, abrasions or other injuries, the cause of death.

The third process of decomposition is adipocere, a rare chemical change in the body's saturated fat, which hydrolyses it, stiffening and swelling it into a waxy compound, a bit like soap. It is sometimes called 'corpse wax' or 'the wax of graveyards'. Basically, the body, or part of it, is preserved, looking as though it is a waxwork.

In the UK, the process of adipocere formation takes about six months – although I have heard of a case just three weeks after death that presumably was aided by the sun's heat and the warmth of maggot infestation.

Adipocere requires damp conditions. In its early stages,

when the fat is hydrolysed into a greasy semi-fluid, the rancid smell is terrible. But, as the process progresses, the fat becomes brittle and paler and when the adipocere is fully formed it is grey and firm.

The phenomenon of adipocere has been documented for many years and it can last literally centuries. Otzi, the Neolithic hunter known as the 'Glacier Man', whose body is on display in Bolzano in the Italian Dolomites, was probably at least partly preserved this way. In the eighteenth century, excavations at the Cimetière des Innocents in Paris allegedly yielded tonnes of adipocere, and it was promptly put to use by the city's soap- and candle-makers. There were some famous cases in the 1970s from Australia where the process perfectly preserved the form if not the contents of divers' bodies found about a year after they drowned due to equipment failure as they explored a deep freshwater lake.

On occasions, adipocere has revealed a cause of death, perfectly reproducing injuries like bullet holes or preserving the fat in certain organs. In general, it is more commonly found in women, the well-nourished and the obese, but conditions have to be right – usually the body must have been submerged in water anaerobically or buried in a damp grave, especially if there is no coffin and especially if the deceased is wearing natural and not synthetic fibres. Its formation can be influenced by the season, the depth of the grave, coffin composition, the soil and the local insect activity.

These three processes of decomposition – putrefaction, mummification and adipocere – are not mutually exclusive. All three could, in theory, be found in different areas of the same body, although that would be extraordinary as each requires such different conditions. But two processes have been found together – and putrefaction is always one of them.

Although it is common now to short-circuit the natural rotting processes I have described by cremation, the traditional place for human remains in this country is the cemetery. Burial tends to delay decomposition. In fact, a body above ground is said to decompose at least four times faster than one buried. Under ground, it probably takes two years for the soft tissues to disappear completely. Tendons, ligaments, hair and nails will be identifiable for some time after that. In about five years the bones are bare and disarticulated but there are often fragments of cartilage and, if I use a high-speed saw to cut the bones of bodies that have been exhumed after five years, there is a wisp of smoke caused by scorched protein still in the marrow and the smell of burning organic matter – something I can also expect from the bones of the recently dead.

The human skeleton is the last part of the body to return to the earth, which, of course, can take a very long time: hominid bones more than 2 million years old have been found in dry parts of the world. Unless preserved anaerobically in a bog, the damp UK climate does not keep bones so well. And eventually, all bones must decompose. Wet soils that hold water hasten this by leaching the calcium and other minerals away. As the bone becomes more porous, the process of disintegration is helped by bacteria, fungi and even plants thrusting their roots inside the cracks and crevices and breaking up the bone more – as well as by gnawing animals.

Throughout their careers, pathologists are approached by the police to examine bones. I asked the attendees if anyone had submitted found bones to a pathologist and two people put up their hands. Usually just one bone is found, sometimes a collection, and they are nearly always from animals. But not always. All pathologists have files labelled 'Old Bones' and every attempt is made to identify these finds. Some bones, like the pelvis or the skull, tell us at a glance whether its owner was male or female. Other bones, and particularly teeth, can tell us the age of the deceased if they were very young or very old. Otherwise, judging age from a skeleton is not a precise science.

For the most part, our 'Old Bones' files remain mysterious. Our main task is to date the bones and discover whether this death, possibly a criminal death, occurred in the last sixty or seventy years, in which case the killer might still be alive. Dating is a specialist skill. Carbon-14 dating only works to a very long time-scale but the atomic bombs of the 1940s, with their release of strontium-90 into the atmosphere, mean it is relatively easy to discover whether bones pre- or post-date these explosions. If they predate the atomic era, the police are seldom interested, although archaeologists might be.

At the end of the talk, most of the officers made a dash for the bar. There was an orchestra of cigarette lighters clicking outside the door. One detective did approach me, however. He was the older man who had been involved with the case of the mummified baby.

'Thanks for that, Doc,' he said. 'I've been haunted by that baby. And by another one, a body which had been sitting in his armchair for almost a year when we found him. I dream about them sometimes. But when you talk about the science of it . . . well, that made me feel a bit better. I even found I could look at the pictures you showed us today.'

This was a rare example of an officer of that era admitting to vulnerabilities. And his words stayed with me. I resolved to redouble my efforts to talk during postmortems. I should not just say whatever came into my head, but present the body in a detached, scientific way which would help onlookers quash the very unscientific emotions they might be feeling.

# 12

Very shortly after that talk came my first defence case.

So far I had only ever been called to a death by the police or the coroner. That meant I was, almost automatically, adopted as an expert witness for the prosecution if charges and a court case followed. Sometimes the pathologist's report alone will satisfy the court, sometimes a court appearance to answer questions is required. The most searching questions, of course, come from the defence barrister.

The defence team will usually call a forensic pathologist too, and they probably will ask for a second post-mortem. On occasions, when a whole group of people is accused of the crime, there may be more defence teams ordering a third, a fourth and even more post-mortems. In these rare cases, all the defence pathologists might perform their post-mortems consecutively, but more usually together, observing each other's work, clustering around the body like moths around a lamp. Then, if we go to the pub afterwards, it looks like a pathology convention. Each pathologist will write a report for the prosecution or for one of the defendants, each report will be used as evidence, each pathologist may be called as an expert witness.

You might assume pathology is such a precise science that all reports on the same body must be identical. This is not the case. Wounds and injuries recorded identically may be interpreted differently. Interpretation can be influenced by many things, especially the information supplied concerning a case: the more information there is, the less likely that conclusions may be erroneous.

So, as the pathologist on call one night, I might be summoned to the scene of a crime by the police and subsequently write a detached, scientific report based on all the evidence at my disposal. This would be used by the Crown Prosecution Service in deciding whether or not to prosecute the alleged killer. I'd probably then have to give my evidence in court for the prosecution. However, if I'd just come off duty when the police's call came, one of my colleagues would attend the scene instead but a few weeks later I might nevertheless find myself working on the same case – for the other side, after a call from the defendant's solicitor.

At the very least, defence lawyers require corroboration of the first pathologist's findings and report. But some defence teams are hoping for more than that. They would like their pathologist to find an error in the original report – which is rare, but still they hope for information which might help exonerate their client. They at least expect a wide-ranging review of alternative explanations or interpretations of the findings and facts.

Defence reports are a normal part of a forensic pathologist's workload, but it takes a while for defence lawyers to learn a newcomer's name, so no defence case came my way for some time. I wasn't sorry. I knew how hard it can be to carry out a post-mortem on a body already examined by another pathologist. I mean, how technically difficult: there will be an inevitable degree of deterioration, whether the body has been frozen or just kept refrigerated; further bruising may appear and wounds may change size; organs are occasionally absent when they have been submitted for another expert opinion and tissues have usually been sent away for analysis. However, all the information the later pathologist needs should be available, whether these are found in colleagues' notes or in the scene-of-crime pictures, reports or tissue samples.

There is another, more personal, reason why defence post-mortems can be a challenge for newcomers trying to make their way in the world of experienced forensic pathologists. That's the fear of taking an opposing view. Our court system thrives on these differences, but they do nothing for relationships within the profession, particularly if you are just a newcomer facing one of the giants of pathology.

Before accepting my first defence case, I checked with trepidation the identity of the prosecution's pathologist. I really hoped I wouldn't find myself reviewing the work of, and perhaps differing in opinion from, some highly esteemed older colleague. To my relief, I learned that the prosecutor's pathologist was one of my contemporaries.

So I went to the mortuary to examine the wounds a seventeen-year-old boy had confessed to inflicting on his father. There were twenty-seven injuries, all of them to the face and head. The skull was broken and the brain extensively injured. The boy's defence team had hoped to persuade the prosecutors that their client was mentally ill. But they had got nowhere and now a murder trial was scheduled at the Old Bailey.

The lad's statement was contradicted by the findings of

the first pathologist. He said he had only struck about four blows while his father slept in bed. The pathologist insisted there had been more than twenty.

When I carried out the second post-mortem, I could not fault the prosecution pathologist's report, which accurately described the father's wounds. However, their varied nature raised some questions.

In a youthful and enthusiastic quest for truth, I set about making a replica of the crowbar the boy had used – except that my crowbar was made of foam. I asked how tall the defendant was and used photos of the scene to stand at approximately the height and angle he had stood to his father. I then spent a long time bashing a pillow with the crowbar: the pillow was standing in for the father's head.

After considerable study, I was able to prove that the lateral motion of the blows would have caused the weapon to rotate on impact, and to bounce. I wrote:

> The multiplicity of injuries can be accounted for by bounce of the end of the crowbar. The post-mortem appearances are entirely consistent with your client's assertion that he struck his father 4 or 5 times.

But my Simpsonian deductions never saw the light of day. A head scan of the young man proved that he had been severely brain damaged in a car accident several years earlier. The plea of guilty to manslaughter with diminished responsibility was now accepted by the prosecution and the boy's trial was withdrawn from the Old Bailey's list.

*

No courage was required to contradict the findings of the prosecution's pathologist for that case. But, beyond cowardice or careerism, is a deeper problem for both defence and prosecution pathologist. Neither party can ever – should ever – admit to being wrong. It is acceptable to admit that there may be other possible conclusions, but, in the absence of any new evidence, the pathologist should be sure enough of his or her view to stick to it.

It was alarming to understand at the beginning of my career that the pathologist is assumed to be right, whichever side he is working for. The day I became a fully qualified forensic pathologist was the day I turned from a not very sure trainee who still probably had a thing or two to learn, into an expert who can never put a foot wrong. Allegedly. So, if you have ever thrilled to the transformation of the insignificant Clark Kent into Superman's invincibility, imagine what a disconcerting experience this must have been for Kent himself. Certainly, I have found the cloak of invincibility placed upon me a heavy burden.

But why is this? Why must I now always be right when it is the human condition to be wrong sometimes? Answer: because the adversarial nature of our criminal justice system has no room for 'perhaps' or 'maybe' or 'possibly'.

Even though I was determined in many areas of my life to follow the lines of Pope my father had given me when I was a young man, and 'speak tho' sure, with seeming Diffidence', the fact was that my job did require me to 'speak tho' sure with complete Confidence'. Any wavering, and defendants might be sent down for crimes they did not commit – or freed when they were guilty.

The greatest test of sureness comes in the witness box.

Court cases (especially at the Old Bailey, which almost reeks of seriousness and importance), can be highly intimidating affairs. I knew that long before I experienced it at first-hand. The collapse of one famous case because the prosecution's forensic pathologist had committed a minor error was a national news story shortly before I qualified. That pathologist's long and distinguished career ended somewhere close to humiliation, not because his small error was even relevant to the trial (and, I fear, not because the defendant was innocent), but because an aggressive defence barrister had exposed a small oversight and used it to undermine the pathologist's competence in the eyes of the jury.

This was disturbing, doubly so when Iain West created his own version of the entire cross-examination for us in the pub, playing both the insinuating barrister and the hapless pathologist for his transfixed but rather glum colleagues.

I found myself recalling this cautionary tale during my first major dust-up in court. I had been summoned by the police to a homicide and, as the pathologist at the scene, I was a witness for the prosecution. The defence ordered a second post-mortem from one of my former professors. He gave a different cause of death. The defending barrister only had to glance at my callow young face and compare it with that of the venerable professor to know his best line of attack. The exchange (recreated here from memory and not transcript) went something like this:

QC: Dr Shepherd, let's be clear here, I am sure it will be of great interest and significance to members of the jury. Can you tell me how long you have actually been practising as a forensic pathologist?

ME: Er . . . well my first actual case was –

QC: By 'practising', I of course mean since the completion of your traineeship.

ME: Two years.

QC: Two years. I see. Are you familiar with the professor of forensic pathology who is also giving evidence at this trial?

ME: Yes, I am.

QC: Really? How do you know him?

ME: He was my professor.

QC: Ah. I see. He taught you. Well, Dr Shepherd, you will, then, be aware that he has been a practising forensic pathologist for forty years.

ME: I . . . I imagine something of that order.

QC: I can assure you that he has been practising for forty years. He taught you. Two years ago. And he feels the cause of death you have given is incorrect. Are you sure you have the knowledge and experience to contradict him?

ME: [*Takes a large gulp.*] I have examined the case fully and . . . er . . . I do not wish to . . . er . . . revise my opinion.

QC: Are you sure about that? You are absolutely sure you know better than your eminent professor?

ME: Um . . . er . . . naturally I respect my colleague's . . . er, opinion. But . . . mine is different. He did . . . er . . . train me in how to . . . um . . . form opinions.

QC: And you are not disconcerted that you have formed an opinion at such variance from the professor you claim to respect so much?

ME: Um . . . no.

QC: Well, Dr Shepherd, I admire your hubris. [*Shakes head with an air of tragedy and turns to the jury.*] Members of the jury, you will, of course, want to come to your own conclusions about Dr Shepherd's knowledge and experience. Or maybe the lack of it.

Ouch! But I don't think my professor had a much easier time giving his evidence: in fact, he was forced to accept that I could be correct. Of course, there was a great deal more evidence beyond the pathology of the case, as the judge reminded the jury during his summing up. They then found the defendant guilty.

I really felt myself to be under pressure giving evidence in that case: pressure to give way on my view of the truth. Afterwards I reviewed my findings and conclusions and I was proud that I had stuck to my interpretation of events. Despite the battering I had received, I was still sure my interpretation was correct. As a result, I convinced myself that the truth was always so clear and that I would always be able to hold on to it so easily, despite attempts to push me this way or that. I still did have a lot to learn.

# 13

My children were now at school but it was well known that I was always disappearing early from the pub after work to take care of them, sometimes even dragging myself away from one of Iain's spellbinding bar soliloquys, because the nanny was going home and Jen was busy at work. My colleagues got into the habit of saying, whenever a case concerning children came into the office, 'Dick loves children, give that one to Dick.' As if there was any similarity between helping a child of my own with reading homework and examining someone else's dead child. No, the truth was that many people avoided child cases if they could.

It did not take me long to learn why. For there is nothing more likely to bring great joy to the private life of the forensic pathologist as a new baby and nothing so likely to bring great misery to his professional life. Fact: it is quite easy to kill a baby, especially a newborn, without anyone being able to prove it. Fact: sometimes it looks as though someone has killed a baby when the death is entirely natural.

A baby case came in, everyone looked at me and I soon found myself at a mortuary on the edge of London. The deceased was a newborn girl found in a black bin bag washed up at the edge of a lake at a beauty spot. The umbilical cord and placenta were still attached.

My examination told me that the baby had certainly been born at full term. She was fully developed, covered in the waxy vernix of the newborn, weighed over 7lb and seemed to have been entirely healthy with no anatomical abnormalities or diseases that could have caused her to die.

The police explained that the mother had been easily located. She was insisting that the baby had been stillborn. The police doubted her word. They wanted to charge her. In fact, they wanted to charge her not with infanticide but with murder. And so we found ourselves in the middle of a really difficult area of both the law and pathology. No wonder the office had been so pleased to hand me this case.

Infanticide is manslaughter, and so carries a far lighter sentence than murder. It was introduced in 1922 for the prosecution of mothers who killed newborns under thirty-five days old. Back then, killing a baby was not considered such a terrible offence as killing an adult. It was believed that no baby could suffer like an adult victim and no baby would be missed like an adult member of the family. And it was well understood that one possible motive was shame at illegitimacy.

We might discount this thinking today, but one important aspect of the 1922 Act has endured. The law recognized that there could be a 'disturbance of a mother's mind which can result from giving birth', something which today we call postnatal depression – or its even more serious sister, puerperal psychosis. This view was retained by a new Infanticide Act in 1938. From then until now, a mother who kills a baby under twelve months old can be charged with infanticide if it can be shown that 'the balance of mind is disturbed by the effects of childbirth or lactation'.

The reform of this law has been debated many times. The Royal College of Psychiatrists recently suggested the definition of infanticide should be broadened to recognize that a baby's birth may have created overwhelming stress, for instance the stress of an extra member of the household where the family is struggling in poverty. Others thought that infanticide was a charge that should equally apply to fathers, and some that it should apply where the victim was under two years old, not one year. Some pointed to a lack of medical evidence to justify the reference to breastfeeding affecting the balance of a mother's mind.

In fact, after reviewing all these suggestions, amendments have been minimal. But the unchanging law masks changing attitudes, including the recognition that children and babies have rights.

As I examined that baby found at the lakeside, the first question I had to ask myself was not whether this was murder or manslaughter but whether the baby had died at all. Because a baby who has never lived cannot die. Nor be killed. And, in the legal sense, a child in the womb has not lived. Anti-abortionists may disagree, but that is the current practicality of the law. The underlying question for the pathologist in such circumstances is: when is a person not a person? And this is important because a person has rights, legal rights to inheritance or title, and human rights. Kill a person and you can be charged with murder or manslaughter. But not if the person never actually lived.

Under English law, a dead newborn is assumed to have been stillborn. If murder or manslaughter is suspected, it is up to the pathologist for the prosecution to prove that the baby lived long enough to establish a separate existence.

One breath is all it takes. Or a movement. Or a pulsation of the umbilical cord which indicates a heartbeat. And the baby must be completely out of the mother's body: a baby born head first, as most are, can theoretically take breaths but still die before the rest of the body is free of the mother. In that case, there has been no separate existence and the baby cannot have been killed.

A baby who has died in the womb in the last day or so of the pregnancy will show the early signs of decomposition, and these are distinctive (for instance, the colour of a dead Caucasian child will probably be pinky-brown). If the baby has been dead for a longer period, diagnosis is even easier: the skull may have collapsed and the skull bones might be overlapping, for instance. But if the baby died less than a day before birth or, much more commonly, during the process of birth, there is of course no decomposition.

If there has been resuscitation, mouth-to-mouth or chest compression, the effects can be marked on a tiny body and this can confuse things still further. A final problem is that the bodies of newborn babies who are killed or born dead are, for complex psychological reasons, often concealed. By the time they are found and the pathologist gets to work, it can be impossible to establish the cause of death, let alone whether the baby ever had a separate existence.

This little girl in the bin bag had been found soon enough to prevent decomposition and too late for resuscitation, so her body was unmarked. So now I had to try to establish whether she had actually breathed in this world or not.

I did carry out the centuries-old flotation test knowing that it had really lost credibility – but fearing I would be criticized if I did not. The belief that if the lungs of a dead newborn float then the baby must have breathed and had a separate existence has been proven a myth. A lung that sinks when placed in water does point to the possibility that the baby has been stillborn because it suggests that the baby did not breathe sufficiently to expand the lungs. But the opposite is even less likely to be true: if the lung floats, that does not mean the child must have breathed spontaneously. It is now known that the lungs of many stillborn babies will float, particularly where there are gases due to early decomposition if the baby has died a day or two before birth.

I also examined microscopically the lungs' tiny air sacs, the alveoli. For what it was worth, the child's lungs floated. Macroscopic and microscopic appearances did strongly suggest that there had been a period of separate existence.

My next job was to read the statements I had been given and see how they related to the baby I had examined. The key statement came from a barman who lived and worked at the same hotel as the baby's twenty-one-year-old mother. It began:

When Mandy came to work at the hotel as assistant manager she seemed all right except that I only had to look at her to think she was pregnant. I have two sisters with children and she certainly looked pregnant to me. This was common knowledge among the bar staff but Mandy always denied it.

The staff all stayed in one part of the hotel and the barman's room was by the fire escape at the back. He woke very early one morning to the sound of a baby crying outside his door. He looked out of his window

. . . and saw the back of Mandy, maybe fifty yards away, going through the gate towards the woods. It was definitely Mandy. I'm not sure what she was wearing and I couldn't say whether she was carrying anything. I wondered where she was going. I started to think about it. I thought she might have a problem so I got dressed and decided to go out and join her. I know people in this trade do sometimes get pissed off and just want to talk.

It took me a few minutes to get dressed. I went down the fire escape and out through the gate into the woods. I walked towards the lake and I saw Mandy walking back from the direction of the lake.

She said, 'What are you doing out here?'

She seemed OK to me as far as I could ascertain. She was fully dressed but for the life of me I can't say what she was wearing. She basically said she was pissed off with everything and everybody. She didn't specify. I sat down with her on a seat facing the lake and we just spoke in general about my girlfriend and the band I play with and other things. We talked about the mist rising off the water. I didn't suspect anything was particularly wrong.

135

She seemed to be her normal self. The only unusual thing she said was, 'I've come on tonight and I've had blood clots.'

I never pursued the point but it seemed a funny thing for her to say to me. We must have talked for about forty-five minutes and I never suspected anything. I never thought any more about the baby I'd heard crying.

We went back to the hotel and she came into my room for a cigarette, then she left. I never noticed anything unusual about her at all. I then went back to bed and had a sleep.

Later that day the staff remarked to each other that Mandy looked slimmer. And the next afternoon, there was a commotion. According to the barman's statement:

I was working in the bar when a woman came in asking for the phone, she had a dog with her. A bit later another member of staff came in, Roger, and he said, 'The Old Bill are over by the lake, a baby's been found.'

When he said this I really came over ill. I remembered hearing this baby cry the previous morning and seeing Mandy by the lake and I suddenly thought it all fitted. I didn't know what to do. I said to Roger, 'I know who it is.'

He said, 'Mandy?'

And I said, 'Yes.'

That is fairly convincing evidence from a witness that the baby had lived, and perhaps lived for a good few minutes if the mother had time to give birth in the hotel toilet (evidence of this was soon found) and then get dressed and walk out of the hotel with her crying baby to dispose of it. And that fitted with the pathological evidence from the lungs that the baby had lived after birth.

But could we say for sure that she had killed her baby – and, if so, how?

This was an upsetting case for everyone, not least because of the cool way the mother had given birth, disposed of her daughter – stillborn or not – and then returned to work that day pretending nothing was wrong. Today she might be regarded as a tragic figure. Thirty years ago, many of those involved in the case saw her as an unnatural, calculating baby-killer. She showed no remorse, saying the baby had been born dead – and she showed no sadness either. The police and Crown Prosecution Service remained adamant that the charge should be murder.

I was very confident from all the evidence that the baby had lived. But then, how had she died? I could not find evidence on the child's body of violence or trauma and no incontrovertible indication of asphyxiation. A very detailed laboratory analysis of the stomach confirmed the baby had taken in water from the lake, but not enough to indicate drowning: it could have got there passively, by non-sinister means.

I gave as cause of death '1a: Lack of care'.

The Crown Prosecution Service pressed ahead with its murder charge but they were dismayed by my findings. They wanted me to say that the mother had taken more active steps to end the child's life.

On the other hand, my report delighted the defence solicitor, who wrote to the CPS:

> We would invite you to consider whether the charge of murder should now be withdrawn, bearing in mind the apparent lack of an alleged act on the part of our client which led to the death of the baby . . . Your pathologist says that death was caused shortly after birth due to an omission on the part of our client. Clearly a charge of murder would not therefore be appropriate . . . [indeed] we invite you to consider that a charge of manslaughter [i.e. infanticide] would not succeed as you would not be able to show that the death of the baby was the result of a grossly negligent omission . . . simple lack of care is not enough [to prove this charge]. Our client told the police how she laid the baby down and rocked it but thought that it was dead.

It is true that the Crown Prosecution Service, for a murder case, had to prove a wilful act of omission: that is, the deliberate failure to provide normal care at birth, such as cutting the cord and keeping the baby warm and fed. It is very hard, in the case of a frightened, inexperienced teenage girl, to prove that not doing these things is wilful. In fact, Mandy was not a teenager and she was not inexperienced, as we were to find out, but, for a while at least, the prosecutors were miserable.

'I am particularly concerned,' their letter to me began, 'regarding the vague nature of your report . . . I am not medically trained but I have a medical dictionary and these are some of the points which have occurred to me . . .'

She listed six detailed points about the baby's death.

Medical dictionaries were the scourge of doctors then – as the internet is now. Sometimes I wonder why I bothered with sixteen years of training when all I needed to do was buy a medical dictionary or learn how to Google. But if a dictionary gave that lawyer a way into my work, then let her consult it: I am only too happy to enlarge on my findings and rarely am given a chance to discuss a case.

In response to these written questions from the CPS, I made a further statement, giving detailed answers to each of her points to show that most of her concerns, like meconium, were routinely found in newborns and none of them meant the baby had necessarily been asphyxiated. I stuck to my view that lack of care had caused the child's death. Although the mother might have actively killed the child, we – I – couldn't prove it.

The CPS were not at all satisfied. At a case conference with counsel, I was put under great pressure to step closer to the prosecution's case than the pathology of the child really allowed. I did not give in. Afterwards, I sent further notes answering points they had raised:

It is not possible to define exactly the passage of time necessary to cause suffocation by blocking the airways, however in a newborn baby the minimum time is unlikely to be more than 15–30 seconds. There were no injuries to the mouth or nose to positively confirm that pressure had been applied to those areas, however such injuries are not always present in cases of suffocation. Their absence, while preventing a positive conclusion, is not completely inconsistent with suffocation having occurred.

I have given the survival period of less than fifteen minutes. I think it is unlikely that the period of survival was as short as one or two minutes, only because the changes in the lungs are well-established. I think it unlikely or very unlikely that a single breath would have resulted in the degree of changes I noted in the lungs. It is certainly the common event that a child will cry after birth but, like all things in medicine, it is not absolute and there is individual variation. The act of crying most certainly assists in the expansion of the lungs.

It is not possible from my examination of the baby to make any specific comment concerning the well-being of the mother. There are, however, no features present on the child to suggest that this may have been an unusually difficult or traumatic delivery.

It is very difficult to define lack of care. In my opinion, minimum care of a child immediately after birth is to wrap it in some sort of material to prevent the baby from cooling. Any other form of care may need previous experience rather than professional training. The minimum care of placing a child in a towel will, very markedly, at least reduce the risk of hypothermia. Hypothermia could have caused the death of this child within fifteen minutes. A child has a very large surface area from which to lose heat and this surface area would have been wet as a result of fluids from delivery, once again increasing heat loss. The cooler the environment in which the child lies, the greater the heat loss.

The pathological features of a huge number of possible reasons for the child's death, including hypothermia, drowning and asphyxiation, may not be present in a child when one would expect them to be in an adult. I cannot exclude or confirm any of them.

The disappointed prosecution still pressed ahead, reluctantly conceding to the lesser charge of infanticide. They also threw in that ancient but rarely brought charge, concealment of a baby.

Mandy was tried at the Old Bailey. Prosecuting counsel was quoted in newspaper reports telling the jury:

When she became pregnant she decided to conceal her pregnancy and the existence of the baby once it was born. She followed the plan through to its logical conclusion by leaving, and allowing or causing, the child to die and disposing of the body by tying it in a black refuse bag. She continued to lie after birth by joining in with the general disapproval expressed when the body was found.

The court was then told that Mandy had initially claimed the pregnancy was a result of a rape but then changed her story. In fact, she had given birth before, on her mother's lavatory two years previously, when the child had been offered for adoption. A second unwanted pregnancy soon afterwards was terminated.

The jury found her guilty of infanticide. The judge thundered, 'You and only you had responsibility for that young child and you failed her . . .' But he added, 'It is clear that you were not at that time entirely responsible for what you did.'

She was sentenced to two years on probation and

ordered to undergo one year of psychiatric treatment. There was a sense of disappointment in the prosecuting team, as everyone knew her sentence would have been harsher if she had been found guilty of murder. For myself, I had no regrets. It would have been unbearable if she had been tried for murder on the basis of evidence produced under pressure but against my conscience.

# 14

Soon afterwards I found myself learning more about truth – although I was now in a very different situation. The prosecution team and I were entirely in accord over this case, and by the time we were in court we all felt confident that we had uncovered the truth.

It was another Sunday morning call-out. More guilt as Jen had to put aside her work to care for the children, meaning she would have to study through the night to make up for lost time. Jen must have asked herself why the dead seemed so much more important in our house than the living and, looking back, I don't blame her. The children were older now and a little more independent, but conflicting demands were causing frequent clashes between their parents. However, our division of labour was clear-cut to me: as the breadwinner, my work had to take priority. Only now can I see from Jen's point of view how frustrating this must have been and how much I must have infuriated her. After all, she wasn't studying for studying's sake but so that one day she would be a doctor and a joint contributor to household income. I entirely failed to appreciate that: I was so work-immersed and so focused on how to make our hectic lives functional that I couldn't, or wouldn't, understand her dissatisfaction.

I set off that sunny morning towards central London, feeling more excited than guilty. I adored my children and a Sunday spent looking after them would be many things: fun, demanding, tiring, fulfilling. But – and this now seems perverse and scarcely believable to me – those pleasures could not compete with the possible intellectual engagement of an interesting post-mortem. Yes, even though I was already a few years into the job, I still could not contain my excitement at each new case that came my way. The stardust that the pages of Keith Simpson's book had sprinkled in my young eyes so long ago was still there. Let other hearts sink on nearing Westminster mortuary: mine beat faster as I thought of the situation, the story, the puzzle of the body awaiting me. And this was despite the fact that I knew the chances were, on a Sunday morning, that I'd be dealing yet again with the consequences of another Saturday night pub brawl.

Westminster mortuary is hidden behind the coroner's court in Horseferry Road in central London, but these are not among that area's famous buildings. In fact, tourists heading towards the Tate hardly notice the beautiful old red-brick court on the corner and they are completely unaware of the mortuary behind it. Like so many institutions of death, it is discreet enough to oblige those who don't wish to be reminded of the inevitable.

In fact, the mortuary had then not long been rebuilt and was the most modern in the UK. Its public entrance was glassy, its lighting was bright, its offices spick and span and its areas for grieving relatives elegantly painted in pastel shades. But, despite all that glass and newness, arriving here on a weekend marked a transition. From family life back across the taboo, into a darker world where, albeit it with jolly staff and warm rooms, death is a way of life.

The smell of the mortuary, death's perfume, in my nostrils, I greeted the small crowd waiting for me: the mortuary staff, a SOCO (scenes of crime officer), a young police constable and two detectives. There was also a police photographer who seemed often to be on call when I was and who was becoming a familiar face.

The kettle on, we went into the tiny staff tea room. It was empty on a Sunday. Detective Inspector Fox spoke first.

'Now then, the deceased is a young bloke. Saturday night, a lot of booze, a bit of cannabis . . .'

So, it was a typical Sunday morning job after all. My heart sank. I'd rather be at home with the kids.

'Had a bit of a run-in with . . .'

Not the first time I'd heard this one either. A knife, bottle, fist?

'. . . his girlfriend, and . . .'

She'd knifed him then, almost certainly. The detective hesitated.

'And so she strangled him.'

I stared at him. That was not the ending I'd expected. Female stranglers are extremely rare, almost non-existent. Looking back now, tens of thousands of post-mortems later, I believe there is no other female strangler in my files.

'Has she confessed?' I asked.

'Turned up outside the police station in the middle of the night with blood, scratches, shirt torn, crying her eyes out. We called an ambulance. She said she'd had a fight with the boyfriend and thought she'd hurt him.'

'How long before?'

'Apparently only minutes. We rushed over there, no

pulse, did everything we could, got him in the ambulance and kept trying but it was no good. When we told her he was dead she was . . . well, it was terrible.'

He looked upset. He'd obviously been in the Met a long time and I wondered why this case was affecting him so much.

'I was interviewing her for hours and she never changed her story. Self-defence. And . . . well . . . she's a sweet young thing.'

His colleague agreed. 'Yeah. Theresa Lazenby, her name is. Nice little face. In tears most of the time.'

The detective inspector nodded. 'Seems such a good kid, it's hard to believe she could have . . . but he was trying to kill her and she had to save her own skin.'

I know how the living send out signals which are designed to appeal to our hearts. I know how easily I personally respond to these signals. The girlfriend's remorse had clearly rubbed off on the detectives and, although she had confessed to a terrible crime, she had somehow won their sympathy. I felt relieved then that the dead can send out no such subtle appeals to our emotions. They can only tell the unadorned truth.

The mortuary assistant handed me a mug of tea and I threw it back and went to the lockers to put on my scrubs, apron and mortuary wellies. As we made our way from the public area to the busy, functional working area, the clangs and clatters of the trolleys grew loud and the smell increased. I glanced at the men around me. For the SOCO this was routine. And the detectives had seen it all before and were nonchalant, or at least keen to appear nonchalant. However, as we passed the bank of fridges and line of trolleys waiting by them, I could see that the young police officer was nervous. PC Northern had not eaten the biscuit the staff had given him with his tea and now his face was pale and hollow. Just before we went through the footbath into the room where forensic post-mortems take place, he blurted out, 'It's my first PM!'

By now my management of onlookers was improving. I could not forget my failure to alleviate the misery of the police officer at that first post-mortem: it seemed to me that he had picked up my tension and this had greatly added to his distress. Since then I had worked hard to appear relaxed. I remembered the Michael Ross post-mortem, where a superintendent had barely been able to control himself in front of very junior staff. After that, I had determined that, when I performed a post-mortem, no one should ever leave the mortuary traumatized.

My only weapon was communication.

'When we look at a dead body,' I told PC Northern, 'we never forget that they were a person once, that there are grieving relatives, that the deceased and their family deserve respect. We're going to help all of them today by trying to find out exactly what happened. We're looking for evidence, we want to help the dead man tell us his story. It's important for all the grieving people that we put aside our own feelings and do a good job for them. So, without uttering a word, the body we're examining today will be our witness and our teacher.'

PC Northern nodded glumly.

I used the kindest, most reassuring tone I could muster. 'Don't worry, I'll talk you through it. It won't be nearly as bad as you think if I explain what I'm doing.'

The worldly wise detective sergeant said, 'You get used to it.'

The detective inspector was determined to be macho:

'Listen, the people in the fridges here are gone, not at home, lad. So just pull yourself together.'

We stepped into the brightly lit room where the body was lying naked, wrapped in a plastic sheet on a metal table.

'He's been ID-ed,' said the SOCO as I opened the sheet.

'What's his name?'

He knew the name but he passed the question to the young policeman, who was glad to stop staring at the body and shuffle busily through his notes.

'Er, Anthony Pearson. Aged, er, twenty-two.'

Anthony Pearson had a mop of blond hair and well-defined features. His eyes were shut. The dead usually look peaceful and without facial expression. Was there a hint of anger about him? Not because he had necessarily died angry but because, out of habit or bad luck, his features fell that way.

I thought then that he was mildly obese – but norms have changed so much that today I would simply describe him as stocky. There were large tattoos as well as bruises on both arms and old scars across his wrists that hinted at a troubled life. The much more recent incisions, defined by lines of blood running across his forearms, confirmed it. Defibrillation marks on his chest were evidence of the resuscitation attempts the officer had described.

Most noticeable of all was his neck. Beneath it the hospital sheet was heavily bloodstained. Across it was a thick, ragged line of blood that had dried after trickling from the side of his mouth.

I nodded to the police photographer, paparazzo to the dead. He lifted his large camera and organized the correct siting of the two large flash guns, the sort often seen outside film premieres. *Snap—flash!*

'OK, that's the whole body, Doc.'

'Close-ups of the neck now, please,' I said.

I was already taking notes on my pro-forma sheets. The ligature mark is a vital piece of evidence and, of course, it can indicate the type of material used. If the ligature is wire, electric cable, string or thin cord then the mark is clear-cut and deep with sharply defined edges. But this mark was highly irregular. Ragged, even. She must have used something soft. Fabric? Perhaps a scarf?

For the photographer's next shot, I rapidly placed a ruler across Anthony's throat so that the photos would confirm the measurements in my report. *Snap—flash!*

I made a note:

Contused and abraded irregular ligature mark across the front of the neck extending from the right angle of the jaw to 2cm lateral to the left angle of the jaw. Level with Adam's apple. Deepest bruising either side of Adam's apple . . .

I checked very carefully all around the neck wound for other relevant marks. I'd seen cases of strangulation where the line of the ligature was surrounded by scratches or bruises, indicating either that the victim was trying to pull the ligature off or, where the ligature mark overlay groups of bruises, that the assailant had attempted manual strangulation before grabbing the ligature. But there was nothing like that here.

'She said she used his tie,' the detective sergeant told me.

The inspector shook his head. He had said it before and he said it again:

'She's only a little slip of a thing.'

'Tiny little girl,' agreed the detective sergeant. 'I suppose if your life's in danger you somehow find the strength.'

I documented in detail the scarring of the wrists, the scratch marks on the back of the left arm and the defibrillation marks, measuring them and defining their location.

'We'll have the tattoos and the wrists, please,' I told the photographer.

He took close-ups of the graphically illustrated tattoos: the cartoon character Top Cat and, on the right upper arm: LOVE. Below it, in larger letters, was HATE.

Since a relative had already identified Anthony, we didn't need the tattoos for that purpose but routinely photographed them anyway. In those days before DNA evidence was used, many a body was identified by tattoos, particularly if early decomposition defied other means.

Although the ligature mark was so significant, I now checked for other indications to confirm Anthony had been asphyxiated. The first tell-tale sign was the redness of the skin on his face, caused by the obstruction of the thin and easily compressed veins in the neck. The arteries serving the brain are much wider and more resilient to pressure and so the blood can still enter the head through them – but, because the veins are obstructed during asphyxiation, it cannot return to the heart. However, the main indicator – whether asphyxiation is the result of choking, suffocation, strangling, or some other cause – is found in and around the eyes. Many, or even most, people develop multiple tiny pinpoints of blood on the conjunctivae, the inner lining of the eyelids, when asphyxiated. These are called petechial haemorrhages: similar pinpoint haemorrhages can also develop, rarely, when someone coughs or sneezes violently. They are less common in suffocation but almost everyone dying of strangulation will show them. As did Anthony. I held his eyes wide open with forceps so that the photographer could see them. *Snap–flash!*

I measured Anthony's height (5'11") and then turned him over so that his back could be photographed. There was a gasp from PC Northern. I felt ashamed for a moment that I'd forgotten him and my intention to steer him through this, but then, I hadn't made a single cut yet. When I looked up, I saw he was staring at Anthony in horror.

'Oh my God, she beat him black and blue!'

I shook my head.

'No, no, that colouration is just one of the normal processes of death.'

He stared at me uncertainly.

'It's called hypostasis. Some people call it lividity. I know it looks like bruising and it can be really alarming the first time you see it. But it's absolutely normal.'

I explained in some detail the science of hypostasis, how it is gravity's pull over the red blood cells after death which creates such shocking purple areas. I also pointed out how forensically valuable it can be. Since the laws of gravity dictate that the staining always shows at the lowest point, it reveals the position the body has lain in after death. But, if the body has been moved to a different position, then an overlapping pattern, like a shadow, will tell the story. Hypostasis can be misleading though. Somebody dying face down, nose pressed into a blanket, will have a livid face with blanching around the nose and mouth: normal hypostasis. It is too easy to assume from this that suffocation has taken place, and I have known many a pathologist fall into this trap.

Now that Anthony lay on his front, I could minutely examine his neck below the hairline. There was no sign of any ligature mark here. Nothing. I called the photographer over to record this and then turned Anthony over again. Here was the mark, right across his throat, and only his throat.

Since I hadn't made a cut yet, PC Northern might have been hoping that by some miracle I wouldn't need to. He had been sufficiently interested in hypostasis to relax, or almost. Then I picked up my trusty PM40, large and heavy. Through my earliest years of performing post-mortems on sudden natural deaths, there had only been its little cousin, the scalpel. As I moved into forensics, the PM40, a knife specifically designed for post-mortems, with bigger, removable blades, had begun to dominate and by now it had long been every pathologist's best friend.

Its handle slipped easily into my palm, its weight felt reassuringly familiar. Suddenly all chat ceased and the tension in the room was almost palpable. I heard PC Northern take a deep breath as if he expected it to be his last for some time. But for me, picking up the PM40 felt good, as though I were a conductor picking up his baton. The orchestra is about to play.

I made my usual first cut, straight down the middle of the chest.

I said, 'We can all see that Anthony was strangled, and we have a statement to that effect, but I have to check that there wasn't some other cause of death. A natural cause, perhaps. A heart problem, for example, or maybe he had a condition that might have made him especially vulnerable. I'll have to examine all his organs to establish that. But first, of course, I'll have to examine the injuries inside the neck, beneath the ligature mark.'

No response from PC Northern.

I carried on working, talking all the time.

'The internal damage caused by strangling may not be very dramatic. Anthony was just twenty-two. At his age, the cartilage in the larynx and around the thyroid is still pliable. In older people, it becomes increasingly calcified and more brittle so it's more likely to be broken during strangulation.'

PC Northern inclined his head in something like a nod. Or was he trying not to retch?

'Strangling has interested pathologists for generations because nobody fully understands the mechanism that causes death,' I continued. 'It was once assumed that victims were asphyxiated. Even today most lay people probably think that constricting the neck simply cuts off the air supply. But we know that asphyxiation alone can't always be the cause because some victims die very quickly from pressure on the neck. In fact, a few die almost instantly, giving no signs of classic asphyxia. And even those who do show those signs have generally died too quickly for lack of oxygen to be the sole cause.'

To my delight, PC Northern's interest in this exceeded, for a few moments, his revulsion at it.

'So how do they die?' he asked weakly.

'Well, we know that compression of the jugular vein – here in the neck – will increase venous pressure in the head to an unbearable extent – that's what turns some victims blue. Pressure on the carotid arteries, here, means the victim will rapidly lose consciousness as blood supply to the brain is cut off. But strangling can also put pressure on the nerves of the neck, which then can affect the parasympathetic nervous system. This controls the bodily processes we don't really think about, like digestion. One of the main nerves in this system is the vagal nerve and you can die instantly from neck pressure, which, via a complicated mechanism, instructs the vagal nerve to simply stop the heart beating. It's a reflex reaction.'

'Is that how Anthony died, then?' asked the police officer, peering at the inside of Anthony's neck.

'His head and neck are congested and there are petechial haemorrhages in his eyes. That suggests asphyxia, or certainly not an instant death.' I leaned over the body. 'A very famous pathologist called Professor Keith Simpson records the example of a soldier at a dance who, lightly and affectionately, tweaked his partner's neck – and then saw her fall down dead. He'd tweaked her parasympathetic nervous system. Ever since then, defendants in strangling cases have tried to argue that they had no intention to kill, they simply took hold of the victim's throat, and the victim's vagal reflex caused them to expire for almost no apparent reason.'

'But Theresa Lazenby used a tie,' one of the detectives pointed out, a little reluctantly I thought. How had she won over these hardnosed men so effectively?

'Looking at the injury, I'd say she used the tie and held it there for quite a while,' I confirmed. 'So if that's her defence, she's on rocky ground.'

'Her defence is that he was trying to kill her,' said the detective.

'Poor kid,' agreed his colleague.

PC Northern, although not participating in this conversation, was still in the room and I'd like to think it was thanks to my reassuring patter that he'd managed to stay so long. He plunged outside only when the mortuary assistant arrived to cut the skull so that I could remove the brain. During this noisy procedure, in which a special saw is used, even the two experienced detectives looked away. Although the SOCO, for whom this was an everyday event, chatted with me over the roar of the saw, it was impossible not to acknowledge, at some deep, instinctive level, the smell of heated bone.

When I had finished the post-mortem, the police officers went back to the station to brief their colleagues and to sign off duty.

'And I'll tell you what we need after that. A pint. Or three. Fancy joining us at the Duck and Ball, Doc?'

I would have enjoyed seeing PC Northern come back to life with a pint but, of course, for Jen's sake, I had to decline. So I headed south. But all the way I had a sense that something wasn't right. I felt uncomfortable. It was like putting your shoes on the wrong feet or your shirt inside out. The Anthony Pearson case was nagging me. Something to do with the girlfriend who had confessed to killing him. Something the police officers had said about her. But whatever it was floated away like thistledown whenever I came close to grasping it. No doubt all would become clearer tomorrow when I wrote up the post-mortem report. And there was no time to think about it now, I could see my own front door. Portal of delusion.

I deluded myself that it was possible to detach my emotions totally from the evidence I daily encountered of man's inhumanity to man. To feel nothing beyond scientific curiosity when confronted by death's manifestation of the madness, the folly, the sadness, the hopelessness, the utter vulnerability of mankind. To be blokeish, the way my colleagues seemed to be. Invincible at work, untouched by the mortuary's vanity fair laying bare all it means to be human, untroubled by any complexity in the concepts of right and wrong. And then, in another one of those Clark Kent moments, to walk through my own front door and turn back into the warm, loving, emotionally supportive, wholly engaged husband and father I thought I was underneath my work persona. So. Deep breath. Stop thinking about what Theresa Lazenby had done to Anthony Pearson and how. Just stop. Key. Door handle. Step. Smile. Be jovial. Ask questions. Cook. Smile. Read stories. Smile. Over supper, talk to Jen about her day, about the work she must do tonight. Don't think about Anthony Pearson, that thin trickle of blood from the side of his mouth, the red, ragged line of the ligature. That's OK then.

The next day at the hospital I took the post-mortem notes out of my briefcase. A smell – broken branches, winter woodland – briefly wafted out with them. The smell of the mortuary.

I handwrote my report for Pam to type. It concluded that Anthony Pearson had no natural illness and gave as cause of death 'Ligature strangulation'. I noted that

> the position and distribution of the bruising of the neck suggests that the assailant was behind the deceased while pressure was applied, and that the ligature was not crossed behind the neck.

I still could not decide what was bothering me about the case but once the report was submitted I quickly forgot about it. I assumed that the Crown Prosecution Service would be contacting me eventually to give evidence at the trial of Theresa Lazenby, and then I would get the file out and start thinking about it again. For the time being, I was too busy.

# 15

I was now proud to be master of my moods, slipping from homicide to home without dropping a stitch. I was also proud to be the smooth comforter and conveyor of information to those present at but repulsed by post-mortems. In fact, I had come to regard myself as a five-star, fully competent controller of emotions. Until I met relatives of the deceased.

Relatives, with their burden of shock, horror, grief. Relatives, looking at me for answers to the often unanswerable ('Did he suffer, Doctor?'). Relatives, wanting to know the truth but greatly fearing the truth. Relatives' emotions filled rooms like a huge and unstable spongy mass, absorbing all the available oxygen, while the relatives themselves sat awkwardly on hard chairs, passing tissues around, mouths open, eyes wet, heads shaking. Waiting for me to speak. Relatives, with their capacity to erupt into anger or hysteria or tears, frankly scared me.

This was something I had to learn to deal with, and the first lesson came, strangely, when a case taught me there was something much worse than relatives. And that was no relatives.

It was winter and I was called to the house of an old lady whose body lay naked and huddled under the table. The police were treating this as a crime scene and it certainly looked as though someone had been searching for valuables: cupboards and drawers were open, their contents spilling everywhere. Some of the lighter furniture had been shoved on its side.

'Cold in here!' I said to the police officer. The weather had warmed up over the last day or so but the large old house was still chilly.

'Damp,' he agreed. 'That makes it colder.'

'Didn't she have the heating on?' I asked.

He shook his head. 'No central heating.'

A detective overheard this.

'Probably intended to light a fire but the intruder must have got in before she had a chance.'

We looked around at the high-ceilinged room. The hearth had been swept and there had been no attempt to start a fire. There was an ancient two-bar electric heater in one corner. It was not plugged in.

I stared again at the fallen shelves, their contents – books, medication, knick-knacks, cards – all over the floor, the small chair on its side, newspapers that had clearly once been piled now smeared unevenly across the rug. I looked at the hunched, defensive body of the woman. She was pitiably thin. The scene was pitiable.

'What do we know about her health?' I asked.

'Nothing yet, Doc.'

'Has anyone spoken to the neighbours?'

'Yeah, they don't know much about her, kept herself to herself. Next door said they thought she was going a bit doolally.'

The police officer nodded. 'The cleaner said she was definitely losing the plot.'

Doolally. Losing the plot. Forgetful. Doesn't know what day it is. So many euphemisms.

In the kitchen, stale bread. An unopened tin of sardines. A tin opener. A jar of marmalade. A bread knife. Curious marks around the lid of the marmalade indicating perhaps that someone had tried to slice it with the bread knife, open it with the tin opener. Letters, most of them circulars or official looking, in the fridge.

No more euphemisms. I said, 'Dementia.'

'Expect she thought the intruder was a long-lost son or something,' said the detective. 'She probably answered the door and threw her arms around him. There's no sign of a break-in, no sign of a scuffle in the hallway.'

'Who found her?' I asked.

'Cleaner.'

'Yeah, she couldn't get in this morning and called us. Said the old girl was one sandwich short of a picnic and didn't realize she was in here: thought she might have wandered.'

'How often does the cleaner come?'

'Once a week but she's just been on holiday for two.'

A scenes of crime officer put his head round the kitchen door.

'OK by us now if you want to move the body, Doc.'

'Got anything much?' the detective asked him.

'Nah, lots of her fingerprints, can't find any prints from the intruder. Must have worn gloves.'

I turned to the detective.

'In my opinion, there was no intruder.'

He blinked at me.

I said, 'Only the cold.'

By now there were four officers in the room. They said nothing.

'I believe she died of hypothermia. I think she may have lost the mental capacity, or maybe even the physical ability, to switch on the heater, let alone light the fire.'

The detective started to shake his head vigorously.

'Now, come on,' he said. 'It's not *that* chilly!'

It is a myth that, in order to die of hypothermia, you have to be outside the house on a mountainside in freezing temperatures. We know that the old and vulnerable (and actually the young and vulnerable) can die indoors in air temperatures that are as high as 10°C – and that even higher temperatures can be lethal if there is a chilling wind outside or a strong draught inside.

If the body's core temperature falls below approximately 32°C then heart rate and blood pressure fall and there is a dulling of consciousness. If the body's temperature falls below about 26°C then death must almost certainly follow, although there is a famous case of someone who reportedly recovered – albeit mutilated by frostbite – from a body temperature of 18°C. (In forensic medicine it is amazing how often you find just one exceptional exception. Followed always by a defence barrister trying to make it sound commonplace.)

Hypothermia is, surprisingly, a not at all unusual cause of death. Its victims may have fallen in the sea or other cold water, or they are drunks who have dropped off to sleep in the park or they are young children who have been neglected. The great majority of victims, however, are elderly. Perhaps they think they cannot afford heating – and perhaps they really cannot – or perhaps physical or mental disability prevents them from switching it on. Sometimes hypothermia is simply the final step in a tragic pattern of depression and apathy towards eating, heating and personal care.

In this case, the homicide team simply refused to believe that no one had broken into the house.

'Look at the state of the place, Doc! God knows what he took, he's gone through everything!'

'And why's she got no clothes on? I'm just hoping you don't find the bastard's interfered with her . . .'

I said, 'I believe she undressed herself.'

'Because she was cold!'

'Come on, Doc!'

'And you think she threw all her own stuff around, I suppose?'

But this looked to me like a classic case of hide-and-die syndrome. The old lady had almost certainly given in to that strange counter-intuitive urge that can arise in those who are dying of cold. They take off their clothes. Survivors have described feeling very hot as their temperature dropped and really thinking that stripping off was a completely sensible thing to do. This is a common response to hypothermia. Less common, but another recognized syndrome, is the way some victims hide. In corners. Under tables. And, in doing so, they frequently pull over furniture or empty the contents of low-level drawers and bookshelves on themselves.

The team was sceptical about hide-and-die syndrome. The detective insisted that I would find evidence of homicide at post-mortem and, in fact, I knew it might be hard to prove my theory. Hypothermia can be difficult to diagnose in a body after death because dying of cold and the cold of the dead can have very similar appearances. Sometimes there are tell-tale external signs, like pinky-brown skin discoloration around the knees and elbow joints in white-skinned people. And the crucial diagnostic finding is the presence of numerous small dark ulcers in the stomach lining.

In this case, to my relief, I found both these clear indicators. Death had certainly been caused by hypothermia. I was pleased to have my theory confirmed but strangely upset by the truth. The old lady, living and dying alone, felt like a caricature of my grandmother and my aunts and their friends, all women whom I remembered living alone in the north of England. When I had holidayed there as a child, the world of older single women had seemed part of a firm structure of friendship, family, community and support. If they could no longer cope alone, they lived in care and remained part of a community. But the deceased woman had lived alone without any such structure. She had effectively died of neglect. Perhaps self-neglect, but still there had been an absence of care – from friends or family or community – which had allowed this to happen. From the pictures on the bureau she seemed to be someone's mother or aunt or grandmother. Where was that someone? Where were these relatives who did not seem to bother themselves about her? Would they care now that she was dead?

I found it hard to cope with the emotions of relatives of the deceased but now, for the first time, I actually wanted to meet a few relatives. I wanted to explain to this woman's children exactly how their mother had died. They made no attempt to contact me. Nor did they show up at the inquest. After gathering further information about the deceased, the coroner gave a verdict of accidental death, accepting my cause of death: Hypothermia with precipitating dementia. There was only me, a junior police officer and the coroner in court to hear this verdict. What a sad and lonely ending to a life that was.

When the next opportunity to meet some bereaved relatives arose, I dreaded it but reminded myself that coping with their emotion was better than contemplating the cruel isolation of the uncared-for. Which didn't entirely eliminate my dread. At the thought of these relatives I felt something like nausea and even considered saying I was too ill to attend. But I knew there was no escape. I would have to engage with the pain of their loss. Which, I now admitted to myself, meant recognizing the resonance of my own, long suppressed pain.

This case was a difficult one. The family's misery was acute because their elder daughter had walked into her fifteen-year-old sister's bedroom one morning to find that the girl had died in the night – for no immediately apparent reason. Alannah had been a keen ballet dancer, sweet-faced and lovely. Her parents and siblings were baffled, shocked, devastated by her death, and their GP, or perhaps the coroner's officer, had therefore arranged for them to see me to discuss it.

I met them in the relatives' room at the mortuary. This had been decorated sympathetically in soft colours. Lighting was subdued and the room was soundproofed from the clangs of trolleys and any inappropriate whistling by the staff. I ran in, the keen young pathologist who had just given a lecture and was shortly scheduled to rush off and carry out another post-mortem, then get home to his children. As I opened the door I was wondering how quickly I could get this over with.

Before me sat one entire family in shock. Mother of the deceased. The deceased's father. Her brother. Her sister. The sheer physical presence of their great grief brought my own life to an abrupt halt. Stop all the clocks.

I desperately wanted to be kind to them. I opened my mouth to speak. And then closed it again. Their suffering was unbearable. I felt it begin to soak into me, like some indelible dye. Misery engulfed me. What kindness could I offer, what could I possibly say? A sob escaped the brother. The sister's head was in her hands. Tears ran down the father's cheeks. Suddenly I wanted to cry with them. And I never cry, never, ever, certainly not since, or perhaps even when, my mother died. I have no recollection of crying as a teenager or as an adult. I have not cried, not once, at the cruelty and sadness that parade endlessly through my professional life. Just ask my wife. I don't cry. But now I wanted to. As if I had to witness someone else's tears in order to unleash my own.

Except, of course, that professionalism required I did nothing of the sort.

So, they waited patiently until I was able to mumble my way through my condolences. Then there was an excruciating silence.

At last someone spoke. It should have been me but it was the deceased girl's mother, a woman whose face revealed her devastation but who retained her composure.

'Are you all right, Doctor?' she asked. Her voice, suffused by grief, was kind and generous. Generous because *she* was looking at *me* with something like compassion.

I assured her, rather shakily, that I was fine.

'Can you . . . can you shed any light on Alannah's death for us?' she prompted.

Of course! That was my role here. She had reminded me. They didn't need me to share their grief. They didn't require my tears for the beautiful daughter taken from them.

Snap. I moved into professional mode. I had a knowledge of their daughter that they lacked; knowledge of how her body worked, of what had happened that terrible night. She had, in effect, spoken to me. Bodies do. An examination tells me so much about the deceased's lifestyle, perhaps even their personality, but most of all about their death. In the case of a homicide, what the deceased says to me, as long as I listen carefully enough, can help bring a perpetrator to justice. In the case of Alannah's death, I could comfort her family with what I had learned from her.

This was certainly not my first meeting with relatives but it was here that I finally understood the obvious. Families who ask to see the pathologist want just one thing. The truth.

Alannah suffered from epilepsy and had been prescribed the appropriate medication. I explained that, as expected, toxicology had established there were no other drugs or alcohol in her blood. Crucially, it had also been established that she had taken the correct amount of medication for her condition. No overdoses, no forgetting. Nor had she been asphyxiated by bedding during a fit.

My external examination ascertained there were no marks on her body indicating a struggle with another person or interference of any kind. My internal examination confirmed there was no congenital heart problem or other obvious cause of death. And there was no evidence that Alannah had died during or after a seizure in the night.

'Then why? Why?' sobbed her father.

I asked them for Alannah's medical history. Of course, I had read it, but I wanted to make sure there was nothing that had slipped through the notes. When they finished speaking, I knew that, in the complete absence of other explanations, the cause of death must be her epilepsy.

Nowadays we know about SUDEP – sudden unexpected death in epilepsy. We know it is something that can happen without warning to those who suffer from epilepsy, usually in the night and not necessarily after a seizure. We still don't exactly know how or why SUDEP occurs – and back then the evidence for SUDEP was even more anecdotal.

So, I could give them this evidence but I couldn't give a detailed explanation of the exact mechanism of Alannah's death. Perhaps faulty electrical wiring in the brain, an electrical discharge or neurone storm that stops the heart? SUDEP is a mystery. They accepted what I said but there were other things they needed to hear.

They needed me to say, 'It wasn't your fault. She took the right medication for her epilepsy in the right doses.' This was the truth. I said it.

They needed me to say, 'She isn't dead because you failed to hear her cry for you in the night.' This was the truth. I said it. And I added, 'It is most unlikely that Alannah cried out at all. But IF she did, and IF you had heard, and IF you had rushed in, *there was still nothing you could have done.*' That phrase is important to so many of the bereaved. One of the normal phases of grieving is guilt. *There was nothing you could have done* won't magically wipe away guilt, but it may allow it to pass more quickly. I hope so.

So that is what I gave them. The truth as I understood it. Unvarnished by phrases designed to save them from it. Beautiful in its simplicity. Unfiltered by the rawness and violence of the emotion a death causes. Allowing myself to become involved in their feelings had added a complication to the truth that could help no one, and I determined never to let it happen again.

I watched as Alannah's sister unwound herself from the strange, defensive contortion she had adopted. The brother stopped sobbing. The father dried his tears. Not for long, perhaps. But somehow the truth seemed to help them.

That interview changed the way I received relatives and, to some extent, took away my horror at dealing with them. I stopped trying to save the bereaved from their misery and now tried to deliver only the truth as kindly as possible – while accepting that the truth is not always simple and singular. It can be a fractured, fragmented beast. I may not see all of it. And truth can be different things when viewed from different viewpoints – which means some families say they want the truth then simply refuse to believe it when it doesn't fit with their preconceptions or expectations.

Not this family, though. But they did have other

questions, and I have been asked those same questions by many families many times since.

The brother, in a low voice, almost whispered, 'What is it like to die?'

Answer: I don't know.

I can comment that, even if it occurs in the most violent of circumstances, death is finally an experience of supreme release and relaxation. Therefore, with no scientific evidence and based purely on my own instincts and my experience of seeing people die in A&E departments and on the wards, I've come to the conclusion that, while few people actually want to die, when it happens, death itself is probably actually pleasurable.

When I said this, the surviving daughter of the family, who had been the one to find her sister's body in the morning, blurted out, 'She looked so peaceful! As if she was having a nice dream!'

I have very often heard that phrase: 'She looked so peaceful!' In fact, the facial expression of the deceased does not, in my view, necessarily mean that death was peaceful. The calm composure of the dead is simply the result of, I believe, the total relaxation of the facial muscles after death. Given the comfort that look of peace can bring the living, this is one truth I distribute economically, although, if asked, I will stick to my policy of honesty. But the dead girl's sister was making a comment, not asking a question. The lines of Pope my father gave me at school came back to me:

'Tis not enough, your counsel still be true,
Blunt truths more mischief than wise falsehoods do.

Death may bring a pleasurable release, but whatever immediately precedes it can, of course, be terrible. Now the girl's father, in a hoarse voice, asked a classic question: 'Did Alannah suffer, Doctor? I hope she didn't suffer for long!'

Pathologists are asked this question so many times. And in answering it, the facts can become very grey as the need to comfort the bereaved stumbles against the hard rock of truth.

Many choose to tell the relatives of those who die in violent circumstances that the patient would have passed out or become unconscious quickly and then died peacefully. Even when they are not sure this is the case. In fact, it is very hard to assess suffering or how long the body can bear it before dying. I can review injuries and diseases and make some guess at the level of pain they would have caused. And I can suggest how long death may take in some circumstances. But, from the body itself, there are seldom absolutely clear indicators of death's speed.

There is a myth that finding a lot of fluid in the lungs – pulmonary oedema – is an indicator of a slow death. This oedema is a common part of the dying process for most people: as the heart beats less and less efficiently, normal physiology means that fluid leaves the blood vessels and fills the lungs. So, people who have their heads chopped off will show no oedema in the lungs at all because their death has been so fast. But the opposite isn't true: a lot of fluid in the lungs does not necessarily point to an agonizingly slow death.

How, then, to answer this family's – any family's – questions about suffering and speed of death? I decided to follow the hunch I had developed into a technique in the post-mortem room: offering knowledge to alleviate painful emotion.

I said, 'Most people misunderstand death. They see it as an instant event. You think that one moment your daughter was alive. And the next . . . gone. But death just isn't like that. Humans only switch off completely, in one moment, like lights, if they're vaporized in a nuclear explosion. In all other circumstances, death is a process.'

*Death is a process.* I've used that phrase so many times now. During this process, each organ of the body shuts down at a different rate according to its own internal cellular metabolism. And then this in turn triggers further processes which eventually lead to the decomposition and natural disposal of the body. Dust to dust.

The simple process of death that many of us recognize from a bedside may last only seconds – or it can last tens of seconds or even minutes. Technically, it lasts hours as the body dies cell by cell. Some cells, skin and bone, can remain 'alive' for as much as a day: these cells continue to metabolize without oxygen until their reserves are finally exhausted. In fact, these cells can be removed and then grown in a laboratory for some days after a body has been certified dead.

For a few hours there might be random heartbeats. Digestion may continue. White blood cells can move independently for up to twelve hours. Muscles may twitch. But that's not life. There may be exhalation. But that's not breathing.

Various definitions try to pin down death, but each definition is a struggle; morally and scientifically. When the individual will never again communicate or deliberately interact with the environment, when he is irreversibly unconscious and unaware of the world and his own existence: that's death. Of course, that may define someone in a deep sleep or under a general anaesthetic – conditions that are reversible. It may also define someone in a coma or persistent vegetative state. But these patients do have heartbeats and show at least some brainstem activity: that's not death.

When there is no heartbeat, no breath, and the ECG shows a flat line, that's real death. Occasionally people have told me that they knew the exact moment, sitting at a bedside, when a relative died. But they are almost certainly wrong. They are referring to the time that breathing and heartbeat stopped. They witnessed a somatic death. Cellular death takes longer.

The bereaved family listened to my explanations without sobbing. There was silence as they tried to knit the knowledge I had shared with them into the particularity of their own, tragic, experience.

'I can't tell you how long it took Alannah to die, but the anecdotal evidence is that sudden unexplained death from epilepsy is swift. I can't tell you how much she suffered but there is no evidence from her body that she suffered at all.'

'She may not even have woken up? She may not have known she was dying?' asked the father hopefully.

The temptation was to agree wholeheartedly. But that would not be entirely truthful.

'We can never know exactly what Alannah experienced. I can only say that there is no evidence of distress. And repeat that death is a process during which life is gradually wrapped up and put aside. And that I believe this to be a pleasurable process.'

The family looked ready to leave the room calm, engaged, relaxed. However, then the father said, to my astonishment, 'It's really helpful to hear all this. But . . . I just can't stand the idea that you've cut my daughter up into pieces.'

At that, the mother, who until now had been so strong and composed, burst into tears.

'We would have liked to have seen her one last time. But we can't! Because you've cut her up!'

The son choked. The surviving daughter's face crumpled. The father started to cry again.

It had never really occurred to me before then that for most people I am the dark figure of death cloaked in Halloween colours who has 'cut up' their loved one. And it was the first time I encountered the false assumption that we pathologists turn beautiful corpses into mangled meat. Although I've met it often since.

Many people – and, I am sorry to say, this includes police officers and sometimes even coroners' officers (who really should know better) – wrongly advise relatives who wish to see a body after post-mortem that they should not do so. Because of 'what the pathologist has done'. People who cannot bear the idea of a post-mortem, even those who are theoretically professionals but who may never have visited a mortuary or seen a body after post-mortem, simply should not impose their own feelings on relatives at such a sensitive time. No doubt they hope to offer support. Instead they can inflict deep and long-lasting scars on those who want and need to say a last goodbye.

The result of this mythology is that, sadly, many relatives who are asked to agree to a post-mortem of their relative will not do so. Of course, they do not always have a choice: if death has been sudden, whether it is natural or accidental, the coronial system will usually take over, and the coroner will certainly demand a post-mortem if homicide is suspected. Society needs to know, and this greater good overrides the relatives' wishes. Bearing in mind that a relative could be – and quite often is – the murderer.

The general horror of post-mortems only became completely clear to me when I read a statement a relative gave following a major disaster. She had learned that a post-mortem had been performed on her son without her knowledge. Since he was a disaster victim she thought the cause of death was already obvious:

> In my view, it was wrong to carry out any unnecessary invasive procedure which disfigured the body and showed lack of respect for it and for my family's emotional and religious needs. To me, he was still my son, and any unnecessary mutilation of his body was an unforgiveable intrusion.

I really do understand that it is hard, very hard, to recognize the finality of death. To understand that the son who was thinking and feeling and animated yesterday is not so today. To comprehend that yesterday he would have been in agony when I inserted my knife but today he cannot feel it at all. And perhaps the hardest thing is to see the insertion of that knife not as an intrusion but an act of respect and, yes, maybe of love.

Here are the words of the QC who was acting for the group of angry, bereaved relatives that included the mother I quoted above:

> The care with which our dead are treated is a mark of how civilized a society we are. Much goes on for understandable reasons behind closed doors. For this reason, there is a special responsibility placed on those entrusted with this work and the authorities who supervise it to ensure that bodies of the dead are treated with the utmost care and respect. That is what bereaved and loved ones are entitled to expect and what society at large demands.

Who cannot agree with him? Except that he was representing relatives who, among other miseries, were angry that their loved ones had undergone a post-mortem.

For me, his words pinpoint why post-mortems are so important. When I perform one, I am thoroughly, efficiently and perceptively delivering to the dead not just 'the utmost care and respect' which a civilized society expects, but love for my fellow man. I am ascertaining the exact cause of death and in doing so it is very distressing to be regarded as a mysterious, cloaked butcher. I sincerely hope that those to whom I have spoken directly, or who have heard my evidence in court about the death of their relative, appreciate that I did my job with care. And, I believe, love for humanity.

Very gently, I tried to help Alannah's sobbing family to understand that her body had not been brutally mutilated at post-mortem but respectfully investigated – for their sake, her sake and society's sake. The world did not shrug its shoulders and say, 'Oh well, there goes another fifteen-year-old girl.' It demanded to know the truth.

I assured them that her body had been faithfully and beautifully restored after this process – as all bodies are – by my colleagues. Mortuary technicians are rightly proud of their skills. Alannah's family should have no fears about seeing her. Indeed, they must do so. Seeing a loved one's body is a way of saying goodbye, recognizing death's finality and celebrating a life.

I made arrangements then and there for them to see Alannah. They thanked me quietly as I left. I knew how long and hard the grief road would be as it unfolded in front of them. Maybe I had made a few steps on it easier for them. For our different reasons, none of us there has probably ever forgotten that meeting.

Of course, I can't personally feel grief for every one of the tens of thousands of people on whom I've carried out post-mortems. Grief is not an emotion I experience as I incise a body. It is something I experience when I see others suffering their own loss, either within the controlled forum of the coroner's court or, more informally, at the mortuary or office. I've come to terms with the need to manage my response now. In the years since that meeting about Alannah I've even come to believe these contacts between pathologists and the deceased's loved ones should be arranged far more often. Information, its very solidity and certainty, can provide not just clarity but support, relief and a sound basis from which relatives might, eventually, move on.

For myself, I would say I have spent a working lifetime respecting and understanding relatives' pain – while trying not to internalize it. Analytical readers will by now be associating my reluctance at the start of my career to meet relatives with the death of my own mother so early in life. And at my subsequent willingness to engage with others' grief they will say, 'Aha! He couldn't allow himself to experience the enormity of grief for his own loss! So, he experiences it again and again in manageable proportions through the grief of others. And, at the end of the meeting, he walks away from it!'

I accept that there is probably something in that theory.

# 16

Although I carry out my work with respect and a sense of loving humanity, I do so with an essential scientific detachment. A few years into my job, I did think I had become rather good at leaving detachment at the door of our house, so I was a bit disappointed at Jen's hints that I was applying it to family life; that the jovial, loving husband I'd thought myself to be was instead a dour and preoccupied workaholic.

Moi? Surely not. So I was caught stabbing the Sunday roast with a series of different knives from different angles while I waited for the oven to warm up. So what? I was convinced I could deduce the exact size and shape of a knife from the injuries inflicted by it and there was no lump of meat so like a human lump of meat as a joint of beef. I'd be a fool not to carry out a little experimentation when I was waiting to shove the beef into the oven. Wouldn't I?

'You mean, Daddy, that you pretended our lunch was a *human person*?' asked Anna, putting down her knife and fork. 'A human person *being killed*?'

'Don't be silly, it obviously isn't a human person,' I said, tucking into my beef briskly.

'My meat's full of stab marks,' added Chris. 'Look!'

I had expected greater loyalty from the other male in the family. I glowered at him over the joint. But it was too late. By now everyone had put down their cutlery.

Our lives were absurdly busy. I tried to get back from work most evenings in time to take over childcare from the nanny and cook the dinner. Jen was now working junior doctor hours. Forget synchronizing diaries, it was a matter of cobbling each week together.

Then, when we were out one day, our house burned down. Not entirely, but enough to mean we had to move out. The fire was either started by an electrical fault, by an aggrieved offender against whom I'd given evidence (as the police suspected), or it was my fault. We never did find out which, but Jen tended to favour the last of these possibilities.

We stayed with friends, we rented accommodation, we fussed over builders, we agonized over whether to sell the house as a burnt-out shell and buy another, or restore it and return. I tried not to regard the house, with its intact structure and black, smoky, largely missing interior, as symbolic of my marriage, but even I could see that the difficulties and pressures of living in a series of temporary homes were not making that marriage any smoother.

What a relief when the holidays arrived. Kids and dogs were all piled into the car and we progressed slowly north up the motorway. Off to the Isle of Man, where my generous in-laws were ready with food, love, parties, towels for the beach, teatime for the children, whisky-and-sodas for the evening. Austin and Maggie were becoming charming caricatures of themselves, he the solid colonial, she with groaning wardrobes of glamorous dresses, the pair of them with more friends than you could fit in the house, perhaps fit on the island.

Jen and I called a truce during those holidays and tension

between us evaporated as Jen's good parents worked hard to ease all our burdens. I was only caught once in the kitchen sticking Maggie's knives into the beef and Maggie was intrigued rather than angry. Then, happy and refreshed, with brown, giggling children in the back seat, buckets of seashells wedged between flip-flops and dogs thumping tails full of sand, we returned to London looking very different from the tight-jawed individuals who had left.

It took about two days for us to revert. And even before we became those busy parents and doctors again, the tensions returned. We didn't have rows: we had seething and we had silences. I was probably trying to make up for a seething or a silence, the cause of which I forget, when I bought Jen a new dress and flourished tickets for the opera. *Tosca*. I was really keen to see it, I knew it would be my sort of evening because a colleague had described *Tosca* as 'a wonderfully forensic opera'.

Such an evening out was very extravagant by our standards and we certainly looked forward to it. The only possible fly in the ointment being that I was on call and hadn't been able to swap this shift with someone else. Sure enough, the babysitter had already arrived and we were in the bedroom getting ready when the phone rang. Jen watched me answer.

'Pam here.' Tough, no-nonsense, organizer of disorganized pathologists Pam. That could mean only one thing. Jen saw my face and her eyes narrowed.

'Right,' Pam said, her habitual way of starting a conversation. 'You've had a call-out. Shocking case. Whole family shot dead in their beds, probably last night but not found until this afternoon. The father survived. Just. Badly wounded, now in hospital.'

That sounded like the kind of case I should go to right away. And my face must have said so. Jen saw it and turned her back on me. The lovely new dress was still on its hanger. Instead of lifting it off, she sadly opened the cupboard and put it away.

'Where?' I asked Pam.

'I'll tell you where, but you're not going tonight.'

I inhaled sharply. I *always* went immediately.

'You got Jen that dress and you bought those tickets and there's no way you're cancelling that.'

Pam always knew everything.

'But –'

'Go running off to some homicide now and she'll never speak to you again! It can wait.'

This was enough to give any forensic pathologist palpitations. The point about rushing to a crime scene is that, quite apart from police urgency and the relatives' need to know, we're at our best when the body's early processes such as cooling and rigor can offer us the most accurate indicators of time of death.

I said, 'Pam, I think I'll have to go because –'

'I've already said you're not going tonight. And if you're worried about time of death, stop. The police already know. The father left a suicide note and the neighbours heard some bangs and said it was about 1 a.m. Anyway, it happened last night and the police have been working on it this afternoon. With three bodies to process and all the other stuff, they won't need you until tomorrow.'

'But –'

'The dead aren't going anywhere and the husband's in hospital so there's no rush.'

There was always a rush!

'Just get there at eight tomorrow morning, it's all arranged.'

'But –'

'Dick. You're not arguing with me, are you?'

Nope. No one argued with Pam.

So we went to the opera and Jen wore the dress and it was a lovely evening except that somehow the family shot in their beds went to the opera with us. I was trying not to think about them but I did. Which body would I start with? How bad were the father's wounds? Had he killed them all and intended to kill himself. But bottled it at the last minute? Or just misjudged the shot? Or had there been a mad, masked intruder who had made him kill the family and write a suicide note – in which case, why had the father been spared?

I didn't go to the call but it had been obvious to Jen that I was more than willing to, and that Pam had stopped me. Jen was monosyllabic while we were out. We returned home and waited until the babysitter had left. And then we had the row. Well, Jen rowed. In the face of her anger I was very, very quiet, like a small mammal crouching in the hedge until the bird of prey flies over. I had somehow managed to ruin our wonderful evening out.

'I can't stand it,' Jen said, 'when you go quiet and moody on me. I'm upset! Why don't you reach out to me? Comfort me?'

Erm. Because . . .

'Is that why you work with corpses, Dick . . . ?'

Now just a minute.

'Because they won't notice when you act completely detached around them?'

Touché!

Although Jen blamed the early death of my mother for my ability to withdraw as soon as the going got tough, I suspected it was more likely because of my father's volcanic tempers. I had depended on him totally and mostly he created a secure, loving world. Which was rocked from time to time by his outbursts. The long-term result is that I barely ever allow myself to loosen the lid of my own volcano.

Of course, I do feel angry or sad or disappointed sometimes. But, instead of displaying it, I retreat into silence. I seldom argue and never shout. Well, I did once, perhaps around this time or a little earlier. Many years later my daughter said at her wedding that she could remember me losing my temper on only one occasion in her entire life (new suit, children, bath, water-pistol). I felt no shame. In fact, I'm quite pleased I managed to lose my temper at all.

Our romantic opera evening wasn't the success I'd hoped for, so I thought I might as well scuttle over to the homicide scene right away. But one look at Jen's face told me this could be grounds for divorce, so I contained myself. However, I was up at 6.30 the next morning, Saturday, getting ready to leave for the murdered family's house. Jen did not wake up. Or seemed not to, anyway.

I arrived at 8 a.m. as instructed by Pam. This was going to be a long, long day. There were still plenty of police around but surprisingly few reporters. Probably they had been and gone. There isn't a homicide – especially a multiple homicide – that is so ghastly it goes unreported. In my experience the worse the better, as far as journalists are concerned. Even today Jack the Ripper's ugly murders continue to make headlines. Only the details of some sexual murders seem to evade the press – although that is probably more to do with information being withheld than a sense of decency towards the bereaved.

When I entered the house of the murdered family, it retained that silence of death I now knew so well, although police officers were still busy and people were chatting. What I found inside was a ghastly parody of the family homes up and down the land that were waking up to a normal Saturday morning.

It was in very good order. There was none of the chaos which can characterize murder scenes: no empty bottles of beer and vodka, no filthy carpets, no decaying kitchens, no blood-filled bathrooms. This was a family which cooked and ate well and took care of themselves and each other.

The teenage daughter's bedroom was clean and pretty, with homework completed and put away by her school bag. Her clothes were neatly folded. She lay in the bed in her shiny pyjamas. A single bullet had passed straight through her head.

In the next room, her older brother lay on his back, shot through the centre of his forehead, from about six inches. Apparently as he slept. There were no signs of a struggle or any other disturbance.

Their mother, a pretty, dark-haired woman, lay on the right-hand side of the marital bed. Hands together as if in prayer beneath her right cheek. Peaceful. The bullet had smashed through her left forehead and a trickle of dried blood ran down her face.

'No doubt about it, the father did it,' said the SOCO.

'How bad are his injuries?' I asked.

The officer had been there much of the night and looked grey-faced and dishevelled.

'Well, apparently he's not going to die.'

I wondered if the father had wanted to die or if merely injuring himself really had been his intention. He'd been very certain about the previous three shots. Had he also shot himself in the head? If so, it would have been hard to be sure of avoiding death. Strange.

I discussed with the photographer what pictures he had taken and then told him what more I needed. I took one final look at the mother and both the children before agreeing with the coroner's officer that these three tragic bodies could be removed to the mortuary.

Once they had gone, and because there were no more fingerprints to be taken, I could wander around the scene and look at it in more detail. At that time, no one had heard of DNA evidence, and forensic science certainly was not as advanced as it is today. The result was behaviour at the scene of a crime that would nowadays be regarded as worse than casual. So, while we were always quite careful not to touch anything other than the body, if a fingerprint taken turned out to belong to a pathologist, then the only result was that we had to buy the SOCO a bottle of whisky.

The post-mortems of the family were straightforward: here, after all, were three healthy people, all of whom had been shot once through the head. Yet it was a most haunting case. That house, with its silent, ordered rooms and incongruous bodies, certainly stayed with me. Its darkness followed me home and I could not quite eliminate it as I closed the door behind me. It was late afternoon and the children were running riotously through the house. The sight of them, laughing and pink-faced, so alive, made me absurdly happy.

I went straight to the desk where Jen was bending over her books and put my arms around her and apologized for being so wrapped up in my work and for being cold and detached at home. Knowing nothing could be worse than the cold detachment of the family whose bodies I had just examined, I whispered in her ear a promise that I would try harder to be a more loving, open, emotional husband.

It later emerged that the father who had shot his own family had not shot himself in the head. His injuries were not life-threatening. As soon as he was discharged from hospital, he was sent straight to a psychiatric unit. A police officer I met later, on another case, told me that it had been easy for the father's defence team to convince everyone that he was deranged enough to be charged with manslaughter with diminished responsibility.

Manslaughter usually results in a lighter sentence than murder, so of course it is preferred by defence teams. And diminished responsibility was often in those days achievable. Later, the 2010 law reforms tightened the definition of diminished responsibility, so that it now can be applied only to those with a recognized medical condition. But for many years before these reforms, the plea of diminished responsibility was fair game for defence counsel and I fear was often abused. In this particular case, however, it did not occur to me, or apparently anyone, that the father could be anything but mad. You'd have to be completely crazy to shoot your family. Wouldn't you?

I assumed the case would end there, but in forensic medicine, despite the fact that patients are certainly dead, cases have a habit of coming back to life. Some months later, I was called to give evidence at the father's trial. I was amazed to find that he had been charged, not with manslaughter after all, but with the murder of his family. The police officer told me quietly that the father had begun a relationship with a female resident in the psychiatric hospital. He had confided to his new lover that he was just pretending to be mad and that in fact family life had been getting on his nerves. He had simply shot his family because he was tired of them.

You might think this is clear evidence of psychiatric disorder but, when the lover passed her information on to the authorities, they immediately initiated in-depth interviews and the result was that he was judged to be of sound mind. The charges were changed to murder. The father was found guilty and given a life sentence. The terrible scene of family destruction in the heart of that house of apparent harmony had been not the result of madness but cold-blooded, intentional and planned homicide.

His trial reminded me of my resolution to be a more caring husband. I don't think anyone, least of all my children, ever accused me of being an uncaring father. I got them ready in the mornings and as soon as I was home from work I was busy with reading, cooking, homework, games, bedtime. But I was definitely slipping in the husband department.

Jen wanted a demonstrative, loving husband. I thought I was demonstrating my love by taking on the lion's share of responsibility for home and childcare during her long training. However, when I thought about the father who had just been jailed, I realized that he might have appeared to take care of his family adequately – while actually silently planning their murders. I realized that it was, in fact, perfectly possible to participate fully in family life while one's mind was somewhere else completely. Did I do the same thing? Was I thinking about work too much while playing the good father? Could this be the reason Jen was complaining? Was she in fact asking for more loving, focused engagement?

I pondered. But I did nothing. We were back to a busyness which seemed to preclude any loving engagement. One of us was always just about to leave for work. And if we were both home there were a thousand topics which required our attention: the children and their schoolwork, difficulties at work, the house repairs . . .

I wondered how I was supposed to fit love into all this? Should I write it in my diary: 'Staff meeting 5 p.m. Love 7 p.m.'? And what was I supposed to do? Bring home flowers? Light candles at meal times? I would have liked to ask other men how they managed to make warmth, humour and this love business a part of their everyday married lives, but such a conversation would not have been acceptable in work circles. In fact, it would have been impossible. We talked about homicide, not love. And so I blundered on.

## 17

The Crown Prosecution Service eventually contacted me about the Anthony Pearson case. His girlfriend, Theresa Lazenby, had been charged with murder and her trial was shortly to take place.

There was a pretrial meeting (a luxury Simpson enjoyed throughout his career but which I have seen disappear in the course of mine) and before it I refreshed my memory with the notes and photographs of the case. Prosecuting counsel had also sent me some more material, including transcripts of Theresa's police interviews.

As I read, I remembered how the detectives who interviewed her had found it hard to connect the strangled body of an adult male with that young woman. How protectively they had spoken about her. I soon began to understand why.

In the interview, Theresa explained that she had known Anthony for five years. She had a four-year-old daughter by him who lived with her parents. She divided her time between the flat she shared with him, where she usually spent her nights, and her parents' house nearby, where she spent her days.

At the time of Anthony's death, Theresa's parents and daughter were away on holiday. She described the day in detail and I can only say that it was a very ordinary day that ended in a very extraordinary way. The juxtaposition of the two was almost surreal. She bought a birthday card for a friend and video-recorded a TV show for her absent family, went to her grandmother's to ask after her grandfather, who was poorly. She tried unsuccessfully to borrow a little to help pay for a holiday she planned with friends in Tenerife. So far, so normal.

Later, she met Anthony at the pub. He was drinking heavily and strangely annoyed with her for arriving early. He did not approve of the holiday ('You slag!') and then demanded money to buy more drinks and then for cannabis.

Theresa borrowed money for Anthony from her occasional boss behind the bar. A complicated evening of drinking, cannabis and anger followed. Theresa herself consumed only one half of lager and no cannabis and her description of events showed her as the appeasing girlfriend of a very erratic and difficult lad. By the time they arrived home with a takeaway pizza, her statement suggested he was out of control:

> I gave him his pizza in the front room and he said he'd lost the cannabis and I said: don't be silly. So I started searching through his pockets and he pushed me away against the wall . . . he threw two glass ashtrays at the wall . . . And I said: you always have to break things. He said: yeah, that's right.
>
> He just freaked out and he started pulling the videos off the mantelpiece and throwing things around, he was shouting and he started pulling the record player apart and I went to hold him to stop him doing it any more (*crying*) and he punched me in the head and I fell

over and I cut my hand (*shows palm of right hand cut*) and there was glass all over the place and I was lying by the sitting room door and he couldn't open it because my head was there so he kept banging my head with the door.

He went into the toilet and he was calling me and so I went in and he cut his arm with a razor blade on purpose . . . I got a towel and I said: don't be silly. I got a towel and put it around his arm, I think it was his right arm, I think he flicked the towel off first. Then he pulled the string out of the light socket . . .

I went in our bedroom and he was throwing more things, my little ornaments. He went into the kitchen. I've got a glass dining table and I said please don't smash it but he picked up some salt and pepper pots and went into the bedroom and threw them out of the window. And he picked up the mirror so I closed the window and I grabbed him and we both fell back on the bed (*sobbing*) and I was holding him.

He cut my arm. I don't know what it was but I moved my arm (*shows right forearm cuts*). I moved my arm and he elbowed me in the stomach. I put my arm over again, he cut and bit my arm (*shows cuts and bruising right upper arm*). I picked up a piece of tie at the side of the bed (*sobbing*), it was on the bedside cabinet on the left side and I just strangled him with it. I didn't want to hurt him, I just wanted to stop him hurting me, I just didn't know, I just didn't want him hurting me any more. I was shouting at him to leave me alone, to get off me. Get off me! Get off me! Then when he stopped hitting me I ran out of the house and came here.

Q: When you were strangling Tony, were you on top of him on the bed, or him on top of you or side by side, which was it?

A: We was near enough side by side. I was on the left side of the bed. I was on my back. He was on my leg below me. I wasn't trapped. He hit me in the stomach a few times, I got the tie around his neck . . . (*sobbing*)

Q: Carry on . . .

A: I crossed the tie over, I pulled it tight to stop him hitting me. I don't know how long for but when he stopped punching me I ran out of the house and ran here.

Q: Did you mean to kill him?

A: (*sobbing*) No, I didn't want to kill him.

Q: Did you think you'd killed him?

A: I knew I'd hurt him because he kept trying to catch his breath. He went purple. His mouth, his tongue, his tongue was sticking out . . . I looked at him. I knew I hurt him. I just had to get out of the house. I had to get here to get help for Tony. I told the man straight away, the policeman.

Theresa went on to say that Tony had assaulted her in the past but, amid much sobbing, that she loved him and felt he needed her. It seemed she was a very young mother – she and Tony must have had the baby when they were still in their teens – trapped in an abusive domestic relationship by her belief that he needed her.

I was moved by her protests, her insistence that this was the first time she had retaliated and then only under immense physical threat from Tony. Sometimes perpetrators seem more like victims, and Theresa was both suffering and remorseful. But the prosecution was planning to rely on my evidence. Which had to be unbiased. So I was determined to adhere to the truth, with its beautiful simplicity, and not allow emotion, with all its treachery, to muddy that simplicity.

The case conference was held in one of the Crown Prosecution Service rooms above the Old Bailey. The courtrooms are majestic and wood-panelled: there is no court in the UK that gives participants more of a sense of justice, its history and importance, than Court 1 of the Old Bailey.

There is nothing majestic, however, about the offices above.

I waited in a room with battered furniture and ill-fitting windows and suddenly counsel, a senior and a junior, burst in. They had come straight from their case in the court below, still wearing their gowns, throwing their wigs on the table, greeting me by name before the more formal proceedings began. The two detectives arrived shortly afterwards. Spending time at a post-mortem together can be a bonding experience and we shook hands warmly like friends.

We sat around a large, scratched table drinking tea from china mugs – barristers didn't do polystyrene – with the various files and photographs spread out before us. All of the Metropolitan Police photographs were put into small folders with stiff brown covers bound by black plastic rings.

I was silent as everyone else discussed Theresa Lazenby's plea. The charge was murder, but they thought it was highly likely that her counsel would offer a plea of guilty to manslaughter with diminished responsibility – which, of course, carried a much shorter sentence. The detectives were keen that this would be accepted. It was obvious that they liked Theresa and that they believed she had acted in self-defence. Indeed, unusually when the defendant has been charged with murder, they had not even objected when she was released on bail.

'Have you read her police interview, Dr Shepherd?' senior counsel asked me.

'Yes.'

'And you've seen the pictures of what he did to her before she grabbed the tie?' asked a detective.

'No, I didn't receive those pictures.'

There was a lot of shuffling and then the barrister produced a folder. The police photo folders I usually saw contained pictures of murder scenes and of post-mortems. This folder was different. From the pages stared a pretty young woman, who was very much alive.

'So,' I said. 'This is Theresa.'

Her youth and health lit up the pictures. She was fresh-faced and her long, red hair was sensibly tied back. Just as the detectives had told me all those months ago, she was rather sweet-looking. A world apart from the usual murder suspect.

I carefully examined each photo while everyone else sipped their tea and chatted. Finally, I looked up.

I said, 'I think . . .'

Then I paused. Was I sure? I did not want to be blinded by any preconceptions of the case into forgetting the horrific consequences of a mistake.

The police officers watched me intently, waiting. The lawyers frowned.

The pause went on too long.

'Yes?' prompted senior counsel in a tone that indicated my hesitation could be jeopardizing the credibility of what I was about to say.

Then I remembered that nagging doubt I had felt on the day of the post-mortem. It was caused, even then, by a dissonance between fact and story. And now I had found another major divergence between the truth and Theresa's version of it.

Yes. I was sure.

I said, 'I think all Theresa's injuries are self-inflicted.'

Counsel for the prosecution gaped at me.

'What?'

'She did all these things to herself.'

His junior colleague reached for the photos.

'Those cuts on her arm. You're saying she made them?'

'I believe so. I do not believe that she killed Anthony Pearson in self-defence because he was attacking her with glass, razors, what have you.'

They exchanged glances.

'You'll say that in court?'

'Yes. I'd like more time to study this case, of course.'

'How . . . ?' The detective inspector was unshockable. But he looked miserable. 'How can you be so sure that Tony Pearson didn't cut her?'

In fact, the injuries in the pictures bore all the classic hallmarks of self-infliction. If you're being attacked, you get out of the way, twist, move, do something: you can't help it. Unless you're being pinned down – which Theresa says she wasn't – or you're immobilized by drugs or alcohol – which she clearly wasn't – then you simply don't let someone slice your skin over and over again in the same direction and in the same place.

And there was further evidence. The wounds were only in the most common sites for self-inflicted injuries (the sites are common because they're easily accessible) and the force used was only moderate. It's not hard to be forceful when you're in a fury and cutting someone else. It's very difficult if you're injuring yourself.

I explained all this.

'These certainly weren't defence injuries,' I said.

The two barristers looked at each other again and then at the police officers. I noticed once more that, although the detectives had charged her with murder, it was clear they liked Theresa. One of them picked up the folder containing her pictures.

'Look at her face. Tony Pearson must have scratched her there,' he said.

I shook my head.

'No. These are fingernail injuries.'

I held a hand up to my own face and mimed scratching it in exactly the same way, in exactly the same place.

'If I remember rightly, the victim's fingernails were bitten down. They were far too short to make these scratches.'

I reached for the post-mortem folder. The notes I had made at the post-mortem were attached and as I moved them the air became lightly scented with that smell, its pungency like snapped elder branches, of the mortuary.

I flicked through the folder rapidly until I found a picture in which Anthony's fingers were clearly visible.

'Yes, he obviously bit his nails. They wouldn't have been sharp enough to inflict the scratches to her face.'

I handed it over. The detectives studied it and passed it to senior counsel, who put on his glasses to peer closely before dropping it in front of junior counsel, who glanced at it with difficulty and then shut the book rapidly.

I picked up the pictures of Theresa.

'On the other hand . . .' I held one up in which her fingers were visible. 'Her nails are cut to a sensible length but she could certainly scratch her own face with them.'

They passed it around. Then there was a silence.

'And the bite mark on her arm?' demanded the first lawyer.

'She could reach her upper arm with her own mouth.'

I demonstrated, not very ably, by biting at my own arm. Then I opened the photo folder again.

'And look carefully, the size of the bite marks indicate a small mouth, too small for a man. We can confirm that by measuring her mouth, of course, but we'd need to get a forensic odontologist to examine her. Bite marks are highly individual.'

There was another silence.

'I did notice in your statement,' I said, turning to the inspector, 'that when Theresa appeared outside the police station you initially called an ambulance. And then –'

'When we examined the injuries, we cancelled it,' he agreed.

'Because you didn't think they were too serious,' I reminded him.

Counsel asked, 'Did you come here today expecting to tell us this?'

'I hadn't seen the pictures. But I certainly intended to tell you that Theresa's version of events could not be true. I knew that when I read the transcript of her interview.'

The prosecution lawyers were looking excited while the police officers were assuming the weary expression of those who suspect they have been duped.

I was confident, at least partly because I had discussed this evidence with my colleagues back at Guy's and we were all in agreement. I knew from the ligature marks that she could not have put the tie right around his neck, crossed it and pulled it tight as she described. The tie did not go right around his neck. It did not cross. It went only across the front of his neck.

I said, 'At first I thought she must have strangled him from behind by pulling on both ends of the tie but she's given this very accurate description of his face as he was being strangled.'

'She did say she was at the front of him.'

'That, at least, I believe. But if she did it in the way she describes then a conscious adult male could have easily stopped her.'

They waited. A detective, his face puzzled, murmured, 'So how . . . ?'

'Tony Pearson was very drunk, not far off three times the legal drink-drive limit for alcohol. Also, he'd smoked cannabis, which would have magnified the effect of the alcohol. The most likely scenario is that he was lying on the bed, incapacitated. I think she must have simply held the tie across the front of his neck and pressed down. And he must have been too drunk to struggle. There's a good case for saying that he was face down, that she ran the tie under his neck and simply pulled back on the two ends. But then she wouldn't have been able to describe his face so accurately as he died.'

The lawyer leaned forward.

'Are you telling us there was no fight in the flat? That she made it all up to justify the fact that she just . . . ?'

'I think there was an argument in the flat – the neighbours heard something, after all – but it was on nothing like the scale she describes. There is no evidence that she was a victim of physical violence and that her action was self-defence. On the contrary, I believe that she must have strangled him when he was unconscious or barely conscious. Then self-inflicted her injuries.'

Everyone looked at everyone else.

'No way do we take manslaughter for this one,' said senior counsel. 'This is murder. And we're not going to let her get away with self-defence either.'

We shook hands and went in our different directions. The trial was scheduled for a few weeks' time and we would next meet in court.

In my earliest court appearances, I had been so nervous that I had only been able to stare back at whichever barrister was asking me questions. Or sometimes, if feeling bold, I'd looked at the judge.

Iain West once came to watch me in the witness box. Afterwards, in the pub, he said, 'So, who needs to believe you and understand your evidence?'

In typical Iain fashion, he answered his own question before I could.

'Not counsel, that's for sure. Counsel knows what

you're going to say, and he knows what he's going to try to make you say. As for the judge, you're not really in the business of convincing him either.'

'The jury.'

Iain nodded his huge head.

'The jury, Dick,' he rasped in his Scottish accent. 'The jury, don't forget the jury.'

Of course, he was right. In court, Iain was in his element. Twelve good citizens and the public and press gallery too was his idea of an audience and he never failed to play to them. I am simply not an actor and could not do courtroom drama any more than I could do emotional, loving husband.

However, I did try to learn from Iain. I studied him in the Old Bailey, how he listened to counsel's question, thought for a moment, turned to face the jury, paused to take a deep breath and place his hands on the edge of the witness box, from which position he could make extravagant gestures, and then replied to the question as though the jury had asked it. His eyes ran constantly over their faces. He delivered his words with aplomb. For the jury, it must have been like having the entire Royal Shakespeare Company in their living room.

There was no way I could emulate Iain's performance, but by the time the Lazenby case came up I was turning to the jury as much as I could. Since I am in court to offer scientific evidence and not to pass judgment, I tried then and try now not to look at the defendant. But in those early years I sometimes failed to control my curiosity. I couldn't resist the urge to see the person accused of the heinous crime whose effects I had witnessed. I was often amazed at how nondescript most murderers seemed. So many looked like that mild-mannered individual you barely notice sitting next to you on the train until he obligingly picks up your ticket if you drop it.

As I stepped up into the witness box in *Regina* v. *Lazenby*, I found myself sneaking a glance at the defendant.

I saw a young woman who, as in the pictures taken immediately after the murder, was pretty, fresh-faced and alert. Her red hair hung in a neat and charming pony-tail. When I gave evidence, her eyes glistened with tears. Her lawyer passed her a tissue. She dabbed at her cheeks and bowed her head. I saw members of the jury stare at her with compassion.

How could this small, delicate woman be one of the UK's very few female stranglers? How could she have carried out this act in cold blood and then had the presence of mind to inflict false injuries all over her body before presenting herself tearfully at the police station? It seemed impossible. I almost doubted my own conclusions.

Nevertheless, I held firm under cross-examination. And I learned later that the pathologist instructed by the defence to review my findings and opinions did not contest my report: he agreed that at least some, or even most, of Theresa's injuries were self-inflicted.

The prosecution was insistent, based on my evidence, that Theresa had simply strangled her boyfriend when he was either unconscious or too incapacitated to struggle against her. All the indications were that Theresa had not needed to defend herself against the extremely drunk Anthony. But it was hard for anyone to believe a woman so sweet and remorseful could have done such a thing unless to save her own life. It was certainly hard for the jury to believe. They accepted her plea of self-defence and found her not guilty.

Theresa's lawyers had successfully persuaded them that the prosecution had failed to prove their case *beyond reasonable doubt*. Beyond reasonable doubt is a high hurdle to jump, but the one that I would want applied if I ever found myself on the wrong side of the dock. Despite this, I was surprised when Theresa walked free from court. I knew that, through me, Anthony Pearson had spoken, but it was also patently clear that the jury had not listened. I felt they had ignored the evidence and their verdict was simply a vote of sympathy for an allegedly abused woman.

Jen raised her eyebrows that evening as I talked about the case extensively and from the heart. I explained how a woman I believed to be a murderer had just walked free. I suspected her youth and beauty were factors in her acquittal, and that seemed unfair.

'Well it makes a change from a pretty young woman being the victim,' Jen pointed out. She was baffled by her unemotional husband's rather emotional response to this court case. Even I was starting to feel uncomfortable at trespassing into an anger zone I usually avoided.

'I'd better pull myself together,' I said. 'I can't get upset like this about every court case that goes the wrong way.'

And, of course, I did pull myself together. The Lazenby case was probably the last time I allowed myself any emotional involvement in the outcome of a trial. It is my job to ascertain the scientific truth. I tell the jury that truth. They have the right to do with it what they will – after all, they hear all the statements and details of a case, which I seldom do. I now desire no further involvement once I have offered the facts.

So, no more emotional payloads for me. No more sneaking a look at the defendant or grilling police officers on the outcome of a trial. Very often I am not informed of the verdict when I've given evidence in a case. If I don't spot reports in the newspaper then I have to ask police officers or other colleagues who might have been involved. After the Lazenby trial I decided never again to ask. I would be indifferent to the verdict and restrict my interest to my own evidence. I must feel no crusading zeal to see perpetrators behind bars and no emotional need for the jury to vindicate my findings. Let Iain West put his heart and soul into his court performances and then suffer personal devastation if the jury found against his evidence. From now on in the witness box I would perfect the art of emotional detachment I had learned in the mortuary.

I told Jen this and she looked sad.

'More detachment,' she said. 'It's your answer to everything.'

'I shouldn't let myself care about verdicts. I'm sure that's right,' I said.

Jen shrugged. 'It was interesting watching you talk about that case with so much passion. Maybe you should do it more often.'

I shuddered. Passion. I certainly didn't want to feel that at all, let alone more often. It was the sort of thing that could get you into a lot of trouble.

# 18

In the late 1980s the UK saw a series of disasters which claimed many lives. Few if any of these disasters could exactly be called an accident. They almost all exposed major systems failures. Or maybe this was a period when post-war values of self-reliance were morphing into conflicting interests of self and state. Certainly, attitudes were changing as the population grew and the systems we relied on had to increase in size and complexity.

In March 1987 the car and passenger ferry *Herald of Free Enterprise* capsized outside the Belgian port of Zeebrugge because the bow door had been left open: 193 passengers and crew died.

In August 1987 Michael Ryan went on a killing spree and shot thirty-one people in Hungerford before killing himself.

In November 1987 a lighted match dropped down through an escalator on the Piccadilly line at King's Cross, causing a fire that claimed the lives of thirty-one people and injured a hundred more.

In July 1988 the Piper Alpha oil rig in the North Sea blew up, killing 167 men.

On 12 December 1988 three trains collided due to signal failure just outside Clapham Junction. Thirty-five passengers died and more than four hundred were injured, sixty-nine of them very severely.

Later that month a bomb planted on a Pan Am jumbo jet exploded over the Scottish town of Lockerbie, killing all 259 people on board and eleven on the ground.

Less than three weeks later, on 8 January 1989, an engine fault developed in a British Midland Boeing 737 which, compounded with pilot error, brought down the plane on the embankment of the M1, just short of the runway at East Midlands Airport. Of 126 people on board, forty-seven died and seventy-four suffered serious injury.

In April 1989 ninety-six Liverpool football fans were crushed to death and more than seven hundred were injured at Hillsborough stadium in Sheffield. It was only in 2016 that a second inquest ruled the victims were unlawfully killed due to gross negligence: the police, ambulance services and safety standards at the stadium were all criticized.

In August 1989 a collision between a pleasure boat and a dredger in the Thames claimed the lives of fifty-one people, most of them under the age of thirty.

Each event shocked the nation. Each resulted eventually in significant improvements, when emotions were calmer and the often multiple, interconnected causes had been unravelled and analysed. Ancient systems were overhauled, the health-and-safety culture blossomed – some might say exploded – employers began to recognize the importance of training, of corporate and state attitudes to risk and responsibility. These areas had suddenly become more serious and security was no longer just a managerial afterthought but a necessity.

I was involved, at emergency or inquiry stage, with

many of these events. Pathology learned a lot from them about how to deal with mass disasters – and so did I. It was the lessons of this watershed era that enabled us to cope efficiently with the terrorist horrors of the 2000s.

For me, the first such case was Hungerford. But this was largely an era of transport disasters, and the first of these I worked on was the Clapham rail crash. A fast passenger train from the south coast, full of commuters, drove through a green light near Clapham Junction and rounded a bend on a Monday morning at 8.10 a.m. – only to find that the slow service from Basingstoke had halted on the same tracks.

An inevitable collision ensued. Because the green signal should have been red, but wasn't. Because a wire was loose. Because the electrician had left it that way. Because he had taken only one day off in the preceding thirteen weeks. And, although his managers thought his work was satisfactory, later investigations showed that it had, in fact, been poor, very poor or simply unsafe for sixteen years. It transpired that no one had supervised or inspected anything he did because he was 'trusted' and because there was no culture of inspection. The fundamental trigger, however, was this: everyone had been rushing to replace the signalling wiring. And why replace the wiring? Because it dated from 1936. And there was a need to ensure greater rail safety. We are now inside a law of nature that sometimes seems to account for the bulk of my work: the law of unforeseen consequences.

At the collision, the fast train buckled to the right and hit a third train on the adjacent rails going the other way. Fortunately, this train was empty, heading back to

Haslemere: the driver saw what was happening ahead of him but had no time to stop. A fourth train, coming up behind the fast train, was travelling at speed but, because the electrical current had automatically shut off after the earlier crashes, it was slowing down and coasting around the bend. The driver managed to apply emergency brakes in time to narrowly avoid a further collision.

The thirty-five people who died were all in the front two coaches of the fast train. These coaches were ripped open on one side. Closest to the point of impact they completely disintegrated. The first senior fire officer on the scene – and the collision had inconveniently occurred in a deep and wooded cutting – looked down and immediately ordered eight more fire engines, eight ambulances and a surgical unit, as well as cutting and lifting equipment to extract trapped passengers.

A disaster plan is all about the victims, but at an initial glance so much of it seems not to be relevant. Traffic and parking may appear to be minor issues, but if these are not immediately controlled rescue vehicles cannot get to or away from the site quickly. The site must be made accessible (in this case, trees and railings were removed), hospitals must be put on alert and the removal of the severely injured co-ordinated. Medical teams must arrive. Casualty centres for the walking wounded must be set up and managed, a casualty collection point must be provided as well as a temporary mortuary. Every passenger must be accounted for and this information must somehow be made available to anxious relatives (there were no mobile phones in 1988). There must be stretcher bearers and people delivering medical supplies to doctors, and the entire operation must be co-ordinated by a forward controller who has established radio links so that rescue workers can communicate.

This is a huge task, and it must be carried out at speed. Speed is only possible after planning and practice. As it happened, 12 December 1988 was the first day the new A&E department at the nearest hospital, St George's in Tooting, was open. The staff who took the initial 'red alert – disaster call' had to be persuaded that the rail disaster was real and not a hoax from colleagues at another hospital.

The total numbers involved in the Clapham rescue were vast: they came from all over London for the London Fire Brigade, the London Ambulance Service, the Metropolitan Police, the British Transport Police, the British Association for Immediate Care (specially trained doctors, mostly GPs, who are on call to leave their day jobs and rush to disasters), British Rail, the London Borough of Wandsworth (fortunately one of the very few local authorities in the country at that time to have its own emergency plan, which was put into immediate action, providing 134 invaluable staff) and, of course, the Salvation Army, who arrived with a mobile canteen to offer physical relief in the form of drinks and food but also psychological relief to rescuers, staff and relatives.

The first role of the emergency services is certainly to take care of the living, to extract the trapped and to get casualties to safety as quickly as possible. Only after that come the dead.

The London Fire Brigade, as first on the scene, having been assured the rail power was off, allowed the traumatized walking wounded to leave the train. They were escorted to casualty centres in the adjacent Emanuel School and the Roundhouse pub and there was a collection point for them in Spencer Park.

Sixty-seven ambulances were used to ferry the wounded to hospital. The thirty-three who died at the scene were removed along with any body parts. Initially they were put in a temporary mortuary but their stay was brief, as it should be. The coroner organized a fleet of undertakers to pick up the bodies and body parts from here. They were to be taken to the mortuary for full identification and autopsy. In any mass disaster, one of the key questions, as well as dealing with the wounded, is: where do we put the dead?

By 1.04 p.m. the last live casualty had been stretchered away from the train. By 3.40 the last body was removed from the wreckage. Unfortunately, no pathologist was sent to the scene so there were no detailed pictures taken of the bodies in situ, which might have helped with identification. And it would certainly have assisted greatly in our analysis of the injuries.

The mortuary chosen to receive the dead was that recently rebuilt and state-of-the-art facility, Westminster.

Four of us from Guy's went, including Iain, who was of course in charge, as well as Pam, to keep us (and the Metropolitan Police) in order. Initially we had no idea how many dead to expect, so we created a flow diagram showing how the bodies would progress through the mortuary. This started with the numbering, labelling and photographing of each body or body part on arrival. Each then went straight into a specific fridge labelled with that unique number.

The four of us, helped by mortuary staff, were working simultaneously, and as soon as one of us was free, the next body, escorted by a police officer, was taken from its fridge and again photographed. This is a crucial part of the 'chain of evidence'. We had to be able to prove that the body that came into the mortuary as Body 23 was the body we examined as 23 and that Body 23 was, eventually, when positively identified to the satisfaction of the coroner, the one released to the undertakers for burial.

Initially we did not carry out full post-mortems but focused on information that might identify the bodies. We described general appearance, any jewellery, clothing or tattoos plus major obvious injuries like missing limbs. The police filled in ID forms. The bodies were fingerprinted and cleaned. They would be removed from their fridges a second time for full post-mortem and for the retention of blood samples.

Identification was, and is, the first priority for the pathologists in any mass disaster – there were many worried relatives, desperate for reliable information. The number of a call centre had been given out through the media for friends and relatives to phone, but it had no queuing system so callers found it to be constantly engaged. One can only wonder at the anger and frustration that caused. But the lesson was learned and call centres were organized and designed differently after that. There were thirty-five deaths but over the ensuing day the call centre took 8,000 calls, and there were many more to hospitals and even mortuaries.

If injuries were slight the police gave information over the phone. Bad news was delivered personally by officers.

It would have been all too easy, without proper care, to tell a woman her husband was dead when he wasn't, or vice versa. For instance, there were four people on the train with exactly the same name. Incredibly, two of them were in one carriage – but only one of them was dead.

Fingerprints and dental records were at that time the only really dependable means of identification: it was no good relying on the loose personal effects like handbags or wallets that arrived with the bodies as these almost invariably turned out to belong to someone other than the individual in that body bag. In addition, the police and fire service were so keen to remove all human tissue that a body bag containing three body parts very often contained the body parts of three different people and not one, as the rescuers must have assumed. There were about sixty separate body parts – heads, legs, jaws, internal organs – and they all had to be matched up. The coroner's staff and the police entered the details onto a database and from this, gradually, complete human beings began to emerge in cyberspace . . . the male, aged about forty-four, six feet tall, slightly overweight, balding, birthmark on right shoulder, travelling in the train's front carriage, eventually turned into a person with a name. We were pleased to reach the point of positive identification. But, of course, at that same point hope ended for friends and family.

We continued working until the small hours of the next morning to get the first view finished. Then we went home to rest in order to avoid fatigue errors before returning early to begin the post-mortems. The bodies of a few people who had died in hospital after the crash were now arriving. These added to our workload but, since these individuals had all been identified by relatives while in hospital, the process was much easier.

Most of the dead at the very front of the train had been killed by severe injuries, not just from the initial impact but by forcible ejection from their seats and hard contact with the unforgiving inside of the carriages. Some died of traumatic asphyxia because the tables they were sitting at were forced back into their abdomens, or because other objects fell onto them. There were many lessons learned from Iain West's overall report of our findings, including the need to anchor seats to the floor and to redesign hard surfaces to lessen their resilience in a collision. There were some calls for seat belts, but this was impractical and has never been implemented on trains. Overall, British Rail, which then controlled the signalling equipment, learned that there were many improvements to be made both to routine safety systems and to crisis systems. If any phoenix rose from the Clapham ashes, it was these improvements.

And for me, there was a personal phoenix too.

The mortuary after the disaster was a busy, focused place and I got on with my job. As I looked at each victim I remembered that they had set off for work one morning and never arrived. Instead they had been crushed and severed, their families bereaved. The ramifications of that would continue for years, if not generations. I thought all this but I could not allow myself to feel it. To feel anything. I knew that the intensity of my emotions was so strong that I could not have worked and so the door on them had to be kept slammed tightly shut.

At one point, I looked up to notice how very white the face was of the police officer who had been at my side for some hours.

I said, 'Do you need a break? You don't look very well.'

He said, 'Doc, I think I'm going to be all right. Because there's one thing keeping me going.'

I waited for him to tell me that a pint at the pub or the embrace of his girlfriend would be his reward.

He said, 'My flying lesson.'

I must have misheard. I thought he'd mentioned something about flying . . .

'Yes, Doc, soon as I finish my shift, I've got a flying lesson.'

I stared at him.

'You fly a plane?' I asked, incredulous. 'That's something I've always wanted to try!' I did not add, '. . . but have never been able to afford.'

Well, hasn't everyone wanted to fly? But the idea of finding the money then fitting flying into my everyday life, slotted somewhere between home, giving lectures, departmental meetings, post-mortems and court appearances . . . well, it seemed barely worth considering.

The officer said, 'I'll tell you, the fresh air up there beats the smell of the mortuary any day.'

I looked around me at the collection of crushed limbs we were now investigating. Did I need anyone to tell me that the clouds are a better place to be?

The policeman said, 'The Met has a flying club, that's how I do it. If you're interested, I reckon you could join, seeing how closely you work with us.'

A few weeks later I found myself at Biggin Hill. Precisely,

at the threshold of runway 2–1. More precisely, inside a two-seater Cessna 152 beside a police officer who was also a qualified flying instructor.

We'd sat with cups of coffee while he briefed me on this, my first lesson, and then, heart beating wildly, fingers shaking with excitement, a buzz in my stomach that felt like raw terror, I opened the throttle and runway 2–1 unspooled before me.

'Pull back gently when we reach fifty knots,' said my instructor. 'Gently!'

I did so and the nose of the plane lifted. There was a heart-halting moment as the rumble of the wheels on the tarmac faded then stopped and suddenly all I could hear was the whoosh of the wind and the noise of the engine. Yes! We were airborne.

We climbed. Up, up. The deep blue horizon shifted further down. I looked at our speed. Seventy-five knots. We passed a cloud. Just flew past it, the way the bus passed me in the mornings when I was about to miss it. I was flying through thin air. In a tiny metal box. And I wasn't falling down.

I realized I had been holding my breath. I exhaled. I inhaled. I dared to look below me. The houses of Greater London were behind us and I could see all the way to the south coast, all the way to Brighton. My eyes rested on the sheer stunning beauty of the countryside laid before me like a feast, like a woman in her finery, like a work of art, a picnic of clouds. I felt elated. I was really flying. I was leaving behind the sad and the drab. Mortuaries full of the still bodies of humans devoid of human spirit, the small failures, the niggling worries, the disappointments, the silences at home, the recent spate of that annoying compromise 'Cause of death: Unascertained'; the idiotic vanities and the frustrating rivalries. All the joyless trivia which can paint life grey had simply disappeared to be replaced by this surge of wild happiness.

I concentrated on the controls of a small plane suspended somewhere over Kent and knew that if flying could make me feel this way, I must never give it up. Ever.

# 19

I gave up flying after five hours of lessons. The fire in our house created such an array of complications and pressures that wild surges of unbounded joy were driven right off the agenda. Spending my very limited spare time alone with an instructor in the air when I should have been spending it with my family began to look downright selfish. So, it was back to PM40s by day and chores by night: cooking, writing up post-mortem reports, phoning builders. Back down to earth.

Not that life was boring. I loved the variety of my work – in one week I might have a suicide by shotgun, a carbon-monoxide poisoning, a drowning, a knife murder, a drug overdose, a variety of sudden natural causes. Each had its own fascination, as long as one detached oneself from the emotional payload death carried for the living who surrounded it. Drug overdoses were still rare, particularly if the user had died with a needle in the arm: that was certainly something to show interested colleagues (today, of course, these cases are simply routine). There was a strong possibility that the deceased, if an intravenous drug user, was HIV positive and so drugs deaths triggered elaborate safety precautions. AIDS was still sufficiently new and unexplained to be terrifying and, in those days of ignorance about its transmission, fear stalked hospital corridors.

Iain West had become the UK's, and perhaps the world's, foremost expert in death by bullet or bomb: his career had peaked alongside IRA activity and his work regularly made headlines. I did appreciate the breadth of the cases I dealt with but colleagues hinted that I, too, should find an area in which to develop special expertise. What, though?

Drugs deaths were a growing trend, so was death by glue-sniffing, but these generally demanded more of toxicologists than forensic pathologists.

Babies? No, thanks. I felt that few pathologists could enjoy working on such morally complex and emotionally draining cases, although in fact this specialization was to explode, in significance and complexity, over the coming years.

My intellectual curiosity drew me towards knives, a method of homicide as old as mankind and one I predicted would last on this planet as long as man does. Or woman. One of the interesting aspects of homicide by knife is that it is very often a woman's weapon of choice. The knife in every kitchen drawer in the land is a murder waiting to happen. And it is easy to use. No training or specialist knowledge is required. Not even much force, really. All that is needed is the ability to get close to the victim. But it was not the domestic or street nature of knife murders that interested me so much as the fact that, increasingly, from the incisions themselves, I often felt I could attempt to reconstruct the events surrounding the homicide. And, although I was coming to terms with the fact that, post-Simpson, the police didn't seem to regard reconstructions as proper evidence and lawyers less and less often had the time or inclination to hear them, I could not entirely abandon the reason I had become a forensic pathologist: to help solve death's puzzle.

I don't think I actively made a decision to be a knife specialist. It just seemed to find me. And my interest was sealed after a call-out on a sunny Sunday autumn morning when I had woken early to see the clear sky and wish, sadly, I could fly a little aeroplane through it. Our burned house was healed and sold, we had passed through the chaos of moving, the new house was in something like order . . . but I knew that taking time out from work and family to continue my flying lessons was still simply out of the question.

The leaves were turning colour as I headed off through the crisp, cold morning towards a village where an elderly man had been found in his kitchen with his throat slashed. As I neared the address I met a line of police cars parked at the roadside. A harassed young constable was trying to persuade a knot of gossiping neighbours to move back.

The old man had lived in one of those big early council houses, detached and built to last from solid black and red brick. The neighbours fell silent as I approached. They listened as I identified myself to the constable, then as he lifted the crime-scene tape and I walked through, they all started to talk at once. In the corner of my eye, I glimpsed someone in a police car. A woman, head in hands.

'I'm the coroner's officer; thanks for coming so quickly,' said a big, red-faced man at the door who I guessed at once was, like many coroner's officers at that time, a former policeman. SOCOs were busy with their evidence bags, and there were a couple of senior detectives. A police photographer arrived.

'That's the daughter,' muttered the coroner's officer, gesturing to the police car in which the woman sat. 'Phoned and couldn't get a reply, rushed straight over . . .'

In the kitchen near the back door, feet stretching to the entrance of the living room, lay the body of an elderly man.

'Mr Joseph Garland. Eighty-two years old,' the coroner's officer murmured in my ear.

Mr Garland lay on his right side. His clothes were bloodstained. Beneath him the kitchen floor was bloodstained. The mat was bloodstained. The cupboards and walls were bloodstained.

He wore pyjamas with a tweed jacket thrown over the top. His hands were bloody. His feet were bare. By the open back door stood a pair of bloody wellington boots.

I could hear the two detectives talking behind me.

'So, they bang on the door or maybe he just sees them outside in his garden. He throws on the jacket, gets into his boots, goes out there and . . . they knife him but he manages to get back into the house, probably reaching for the phone . . .'

I looked back at Mr Garland. The bloodstaining was unusually distributed. His jacket and pyjamas were heavily stained on the front. Confusingly, the blood extended down to the upper calf. There was no blood below this except on the soles of his feet. The wellington boots, however, were bloodstained on the outside and in a narrow rim on the inside at the top.

It was obvious that he had been wearing the wellies at

or after the time he received the injuries. Then he had taken them off when he came into the house. They stood neatly in what was almost certainly their accustomed place by the door. Their owner probably had a long-practised, ingrained habit of stepping out of them as he entered.

'I bet he once had a wife who nagged him about bringing mud onto the kitchen floor,' I said to no one in particular.

I stared out into the back garden, which was being combed now by a number of police officers. I saw a trail of blood leading to the greenhouse. Outside it, Mr Garland's pots were stacked. Inside, through dirty windows, the summer's tomato plants were visible. They were brown, dying off as autumn closed in.

Beyond the greenhouse was a garage and parking area. A deep pool of blood was visible in the parking area: clearly the wound had been inflicted here. A red car stood nearby at an odd angle, the driver's door not properly shut, as if someone had leapt out in a hurry.

'It's the daughter's,' explained the coroner's officer.

The photographer had finished his initial work now and I went back to the body. I rolled Mr Garland over and a huge incised wound on the side of his neck, just above the jacket, gaped at me. A knife had cut through the muscles and the right jugular vein and partially severed the carotid artery. There were a number of other horizontal wounds across the throat, but none so deep as the wound that had most certainly killed him.

I felt his arms and legs. Rigor mortis had set in but was not fully established in the legs. I took his temperature.

Another policeman was listening intently to his radio.

'Suspicious van . . . two men, early twenties, approached a pensioner this morning. Asked if he had any gardening work. The van was a white Ford, registration probably included letters T and K . . .'

'Get someone out there looking for it,' said a senior voice, who then introduced himself to me as a detective superintendent.

I had been crouching by the body and stood up now.

'Could you ask his daughter if he was left-handed?'

The super looked at me for a moment and then disappeared to the police car. Through the open door I heard Mr Garland's tearful daughter confirm that he was indeed left-handed. She knew what this question meant, even perhaps before the detective, because she began to wail.

'I don't think this is a murder investigation,' I said when the detective came back.

The officers, busy around the scene, inside and out, all seemed to freeze.

'This wound is self-inflicted. I'm afraid Mr Garland killed himself.'

The super shook his head.

'That was our first thought. But we've searched high and low for a knife and there just isn't one.'

'There must be.'

The detective began to look annoyed: 'You can't kill yourself and then dispose of the weapon. There's no weapon here. This is a homicide.'

'Maybe he dropped the knife into the bushes.'

The super gestured to his team of officers, even now busy in the flower beds.

'This is their second sweep of the garden. It's not that big and there's no knife.'

I was sure the knife was there. I was sure the old man had killed himself. I paused and considered. How sure was I?

The detective was glaring at me. 'You don't know anything until you do the post-mortem, Doc.'

People always think that by opening the bodies of the dead I will find their secrets locked inside, like someone who cracks safes. But in this case, I already knew a great deal from careful study of the body's external appearance.

There was no point in arguing, as I would have to do a post-mortem anyway. I turned back to the coroner's officer. 'Can you arrange to take him to a mortuary now?'

He nodded and called over two uniformed police officers.

'Right, let's get him bagged up and over to the Royal Surrey.'

I turned back to the super. I was confident.

'Of course, I'll do the post-mortem, but I'm sure this is a suicide.'

'What makes you so sure?' he asked me, and not pleasantly. It was a tone I knew already but I'd rarely encountered it at the scene of a crime, where there is generally quiet, good-natured teamwork. No, that sneer belonged in court, employed by a senior defence barrister setting out to humiliate a pathologist whose evidence inconveniences his client.

I responded in my most clinical voice.

'First, the site of the injury. Mr Garland has cut himself

several times, and the site he's chosen is absolutely typical of self-inflicted incisions. They're nearly always on the neck or the wrists. He cut the right side of the neck, which would be most unlikely if he was right-handed. But you've just confirmed that he was left-handed. And look at all those smaller injuries. They're parallel.'

The detective glanced, reluctantly, at the old man's neck. I pointed to the thin, superficial lines of blood on either side of the large slash wound and explained hesitation injuries to him. 'We don't know exactly why people do this: perhaps they're just building up their courage. Preparing for the pain. Or trying to find the right place. But hesitation injuries are strong indicators of suicide.'

The detective still looked sceptical.

'Those lines *always* mean it's suicide?'

'In my experience that is usually the case.' My experience at the time was not so very extensive, but I didn't plan to tell the officer that.

'If he cut himself out there . . .' The detective indicated the pool of thick blood in the parking area. '. . . and died just here, how much time would he have had to dispose of the knife?'

I thought.

'Up to a minute.'

Not that he would have been able to hide the knife after losing all that blood. He might have been able to throw it but he had almost certainly just dropped it.

The detective, who really seemed to want a homicide to brighten up his Sunday, said, 'Someone could have knifed him and run off with the weapon.'

'Well . . .'

223

'It's possible, you admit the possibility, that his wound was inflicted by someone else?'

I hesitated. Of course it was possible, anything was possible. But it was my job to collect and present evidence, not to speculate on every wild theory.

I said, 'It's unlikely. But it's possible.'

The detective looked triumphant.

'However, I believe that the knife must be here,' I said. 'And in a fairly obvious place.'

The team looking for the knife heard this. They paused. Some put their hands on their hips, others stood straight, staring at me. They had been searching for a while now and didn't want to hear they had missed something obvious.

I went out through the little back door, past the bloody wellington boots, past the greenhouse and the old clay flowerpots, past an ancient tin bath that lay on its side, following the blood trail to its source.

'He lost a lot of blood and he was losing more fast as he moved back towards the house, I really think he would have just dropped the knife somewhere near this spot rather than throwing it,' I said. 'Perhaps the daughter . . . ?'

'Says she hasn't touched a thing.'

When there is a suicide, often a relative or friend suspects it has taken place. Perhaps Mr Garland had threatened suicide or maybe he had just seemed very depressed. I tried to imagine the middle-aged daughter arriving at speed in her red car, heart beating, scared of what she might find. The first thing she would have seen was the pool of blood. Her car had screeched to a halt just short of it, and, leaving the vehicle askew across the parking area, barely even shutting the door, she would have jumped out and run into the house to find her father.

'No knife, no suicide,' stated the detective firmly.

'Could you reverse her car, please?'

Everyone looked at everyone else and the detective went to ask the daughter for the keys, then came out and slowly backed the car away from the parking area.

Beneath the wheel's original position lay a bloody, bone-handled bread knife.

The detective can have had no idea of the relief I felt at having my theory confirmed. I had probably sounded very sure of myself. And I was very sure. But deep down I have, since childhood, recognized that life is a series of unexpected twists and turns. This knowledge enslaves me. Although it is my job to be certain, I was unable that day, and am still unable, to escape a greater certainty: that there are always other possibilities.

## 20

By now I was beginning to suspect that my attempts to reconstruct homicides from the track of stab wounds might just be eclipsed by a technique which had recently appeared on the distant periphery of forensic work. People had started to talk about DNA testing. DNA, they said, would be a better means of identification than fingerprinting or any of our other current methods. We discussed it in the pub during one of our raucous office Friday lunchtimes, our debate leaking into the afternoon, the secretaries and technicians all joining in. Was DNA the future? Or one of those technological advances which would have no workable application for years and years?

The new developments did make me wonder if my special interest in the track of stab wounds would soon be so old-fashioned it would help no one. My fascination with the idea did not abate but it happened that at around that time another specialization seemed to find me. At first I tried to ignore it, but somehow it managed to kick me hard in a vulnerable place I scarcely knew I had: my social conscience. I did think I already worked for society: forensic pathologists helped families and the state to understand the dead and so find justice, didn't they? I was rather slow to take on board the idea that I personally might have a more direct role to play in bringing about social change.

Working closely with the police at the scene of a crime was a part of my job. Their professionalism and camaraderie made the chaos, blood, filth and human tragedy of the average homicide a lot easier to deal with. When I had a good relationship with the officers involved they sometimes kept me informed as their investigations progressed, and I valued that.

How hard it was, then, to bear witness to another sort of policing. One that had little in common with the dignified, serious men and women I encountered.

On arriving at a hospital mortuary for a post-mortem one night, the information I was given at the briefing was a bit sketchy. I soon gathered why. The patient had died while in the care of the prison system. I noticed that there was no banter or small talk as we changed and walked into the post-mortem room to examine the body.

The deceased was a twenty-eight-year-old Nigerian. An external examination revealed abrasions on the front of his nose and around the lips. I saw he had recent bruising to his arms and particularly around his wrists, as well as on his abdomen.

I said, 'So was he wearing a body belt when he died?'

They nodded glumly.

A body belt is an unattractive contraption consisting of a thick, heavy, leather belt with handcuffs passing through a ring on each side. The belt, of course, goes around the abdomen and the wrists are attached to it by the handcuffs.

When I examined the deceased internally I found that he had severe atheroma (furring up of the arteries) but only in one place: inside a carotid artery, the main artery in the neck that takes blood to the brain: very unusual in a twenty-eight-year-old. In a few years' time that might well have become life threatening. But it certainly did not cause his death.

Further tests showed that he also had sickle-cell trait.

Sickle-cell disease is the UK's fastest growing genetic disorder. It is carried by millions of people worldwide, mostly of African or Caribbean origin. Those who suffer from it are more likely to survive malaria (not very useful in metropolitan London). But that's the end of the good news. It is caused by a mutation in the haemoglobin gene and haemoglobin's vital function is to transport oxygen around the body. In healthy individuals with normal haemoglobin, these red blood cells are fat and round with a dimple in the middle – not unlike a ring doughnut. And, most importantly, they are bendy. The sickle-cell genetic mutation swaps one amino acid and this means that the haemoglobin folds differently. For most of the time that's not a problem but when the haemoglobin molecule is not holding on to an oxygen molecule it can become stiff and fixed in an unusual shape. In this case, red blood cells can look like odd bananas – or sickles, hence the name of the disease. The result of the stiffness and strange shape is that, instead of flowing smoothly through the blood vessels, the blood cells tend to pile up, interlock and block the vessels – starving vital organs of oxygen.

Pains in the joints and abdomen and often anaemia are just the start of the problems these blockages can cause. Sufferers were once virtually guaranteed a short life but increasing knowledge of the disease and new drug treatments are changing all that, and maybe gene therapy will soon be available to help further.

The full, severe, disease means that the individual has inherited the same faulty gene from both parents. This is called homozygous and, as a result, sufferers can only make the faulty haemoglobin. However, inherit one faulty gene from one parent and one normal gene from the other and sufferers are called heterozygous. They can make some normal haemoglobin as well as some faulty haemoglobin. These individuals will have the lesser form of the disease, which, not surprisingly in a genetic disorder of this sort, is even more widespread than full sickle-cell disease. This is called sickle-cell trait.

Sickle-cell trait was for a long time thought to have no significant impact on those who had it (unless they caught malaria). Only in recent decades has it been recognized as a major risk factor in certain circumstances. And those are circumstances that in any way significantly deprive sufferers of oxygen. So, no climbing Everest for those with sickle-cell trait. In fact, sickle-cell trait sufferers should avoid all situations where there may be any threat of oxygen deprivation at all, so as well as climbing high mountains, that includes scuba diving, parachuting . . . and being forcefully restrained. Of course, the former are a matter of choice. But not the latter.

This was the first case for me, although soon others followed, in which a black patient died under restraint and in whom I could find only a few sickle cells in the tissues when I looked down the microscope. This indicated that they did not have full sickle-cell disease but sickle-cell trait, and this could then be confirmed by specialist tests on their haemoglobin. Sadly, many probably did not even know that they were carriers.

This particular patient also showed signs of hypoxia, which is a lack of oxygen. He had been forcibly restrained but none of his injuries was actually life threatening. Clearly, then, the police actions must have gone further than was indicated by the areas of bruising, all of which I noted carefully in my report.

It was only later that I was given the full story. He was being held at a London jail awaiting trial for conspiracy to defraud. I'm not sure what he did for his behaviour to be described by prison medical officers as 'strange' enough for them to arrange his transfer to the hospital wing of Brixton jail. I think from that I would assume mental health problems, although none of the medical notes specifically said so. I didn't think that this behaviour was drug-related since, although cocaine was found in his urine, it was very minimal.

During transportation to the hospital wing at Brixton he became 'agitated or aggressive, then unresponsive'. That description comes from notes taken by the doctor at the accident and emergency department when the patient was driven there later. According to the police's own records, on arrival at Brixton Prison's hospital wing 'it was noticed that he appeared not to be breathing'.

So he was bundled into the back of a van and taken to A&E. He was given CPR on the way but those resuscitation attempts were not successful. In fact, the A&E doctor's notes added, 'fingers stiff!'

It seemed to me that he may have been held in a way that restricted his breathing and his oxygen supply – possibly face down, or maybe someone knelt on his chest.

But the post-mortem showed that death was caused primarily by the fact that he had severe pneumonia.

This was enough to slip him out of the suspicious death category. He had died from natural causes – a combination of pneumonia and sickle-cell trait. Although I felt and said that he might have survived pneumonia if he had been given proper treatment immediately and if he had not been restrained in a body belt face down, or in some other position that further restricted his ability to breathe.

The deceased was of no fixed abode and he may, therefore, have been living rough and contracted pneumonia before his arrest, or he may actually have contracted it in custody. An inquest was held and a verdict of death by natural causes was given – aggravated, the coroner said in something of an understatement, by lack of care.

This took place less than thirty years ago but in those days in general – and this is not true of all communities – the bulk of society thought criminals deserved what they got, and that the police were always, or at least usually, right. So, even without the natural and mitigating factors of his sickle-cell trait and pneumonia, there would have been no outcry at the death of a prisoner. And I am sorry to say that, the times being what they were, such indifference was especially true if the prisoner was black.

Indifference from both public and police meant there was an almost total lack of training and understanding about how and when to restrain someone safely. Such training was not considered relevant or useful for the day-to-day work of a policeman or prison officer. It was acceptable for staff simply to rugby-tackle people, jump on them, wrestle with them, do whatever was necessary to get them under control – and 'control' meant 'still'.

Police and prison officers were trusted to do what was right and the nation was uncaring about the possibility that they might not. I, however, could not share this attitude. I saw a series of deaths in custody or under restraint. Many of the dead were black. This was not just a sickle-cell problem, although it was sickle-cell that had brought it to my attention. I felt that I had to do something. But what? I worked with the Met and good, supportive relations were essential at the scene of a crime and afterwards. I liked and respected many officers. A pleasant working relationship with them was essential to me and so I did not know how to call them on their behaviour. But I knew I had to, and as the deaths under restraint were more than occasional, I realized that I had to focus on this. I just wasn't sure yet how to use my knowledge to improve the situation. After all, pathologists examine bodies and understand the cause of death. Our findings might contribute to the saving of future lives or the process of justice. But it wasn't my job to change the world. Was it?

## 21

I could not ignore the problem of death caused by restraint but, intellectually and analytically, I remained committed to studying knife murders. As a bullets-and-bombs man, Iain West had specialized in a comparatively straightforward area. The perpetrators want someone dead and they shoot them, end of story. Stab wounds require perpetrator and victim to be up close and personal. Stab wounds often involve mixed motives. Stab wounds may have more to do with a sense of theatre than a definite wish to kill – particularly if the injuries are self-inflicted. But what really interested me was my theory that every wound track tells a story. I was still sure that the exact track a knife made into the body – and often victims are stabbed many times – could provide a sort of photograph of the homicide itself if one knew enough about wounding.

At each knife murder I was anxious to learn anything I could from the wounds. Very soon after the suicide of the old man with the bread knife came another death by knife. It was an entirely routine homicide but it did show me that all those experiments with the Sunday roast were getting me somewhere.

Winter followed quickly behind that sunny autumn day, and soon the first frost came. One morning, I was called to a body found by a canal in north London. I arrived at noon to find a young man in jeans and jacket lying face down in a grassy waste area, his arms beneath him. The temperature was still only 2°C and this did not help the usual problems determining the time of death. Body temperature was down to 20°C and the police photographs showed that there was frost still on the body when found. Rigor mortis was established but not fully fixed.

All I could tell the police from this was that death had occurred at some time between midnight and 6 a.m. – eliciting the usual response of veiled frustration.

The grass adjacent to the deceased's feet was bloodstained and next to the body was a bloodstained kitchen knife. I turned him over and saw that the mouth, nose, hand and front of the chest were covered in blood.

We moved him to the mortuary for a full post-mortem, where I confirmed that a single stab wound had penetrated first his clothes, then the cartilage of three adjacent ribs. The cartilage had deflected the blade. Just a little, but that small deflection meant sadly that the knife went straight into the aorta. It had cut through the aorta to the trachea behind it. The track ended in the oesophagus. The total track length from the skin surface was 12cm. The incision went horizontally from front to back and slightly from right to left.

The black-handled kitchen knife found nearby would certainly have been the right size and shape to cause this wound. The force used must have been more than moderate as it had cut through both clothing and the three ribs. There were also minor abrasions on the deceased's face and various abrasions on the left arm.

It looked like a straightforward stabbing. The police were trying to match it to the defendant's story. The defendant and victim, both aged about twenty, had been drinking together and then went out for a walk. They were good friends but, as revealed during his police interview, the accused was secretly angry with his mate:

Q: What did you talk about?
A: Nothing really.
Q: Were you armed?
A: No.
Q: Was he?
A: Yeah, he always carries a knife.
Q: On previous occasions have you both carried knives?
A: Yeah, but mine was at home then.
Q: I must tell you that you are still under caution. Do you know how he died?
A: I think I do.
Q: Please tell us.
A: We reached the canal and he said he felt sick. So I stood there and waited for him and I looked down and saw my trainer was undone so I bent down to retie my lace and he said, what do you think of me going out with your sister?
Q: Mary?
A: Yes.
Q: How old is Mary?
A: Thirteen.
Q: What did you say?
A: I said I didn't like it very much because she's only thirteen. I looked up to face him and ask him why he was asking but I didn't have time, he was drawing something from his clothing. I thought he was

going to hit me. So I panic and I push him then I turn and run. I turned round once and saw him stumbling backwards. I carried on running. I didn't know he was hurt or I would have gone back and helped him.

Further questioning revealed how upset the young man was at the possibility that his friend was having sex with the thirteen-year-old Mary. After one of many breaks, during which he conferred with his solicitor, the accused said, 'If it's the knife I think it is then I saw that in his flat. It had fallen out of the plate rack with a load of others and I picked it up and put it on the worktop.'

The solicitor later asked once again for a few words alone with his client who, on re-emerging, admitted to causing the death – but insisted it had been an accident: 'He was my best friend and no way did I mean to hurt him, that's it.'

I was sure that the defendant's version of events was false. My own instinct told me that it would not be possible to turn around a knife held by someone else and penetrate the chest with it in this way – the wound was straight and horizontal. And certainly not to penetrate so high into the chest from a low, crouching position.

However, on the basis that the defendant was innocent until proven guilty, I tried re-enacting the scene at home. I crouched on the floor pretending to tie my shoelace (with my right hand), look up, and deflect an assailant's approaching ruler (standing in for the knife – which I held in my left hand) into the assailant (a pillow on a chair) and cause a horizontal, straight wound. I had just got the ruler into the pillow when I realized that someone else was in the room.

I turned around. Chris had come into the study. Both children had been taught to knock so that they wouldn't stumble upon any upsetting material. I must have been so engrossed that I didn't hear him. Now he was staring at me rather awkwardly.

'Yes?' I said, trying to look as if this was all perfectly normal.

He was clutching a schoolbook.

'What are you doing?' he asked in a voice which required some explanation. He was nine now and a relaxed, even-tempered child who seemed in no way related to the screaming baby emperor who had tortured us for nights on end.

I stood up. Honesty was probably the best policy.

'Well, I'm trying to see if a man tying his shoelace . . . that's me, here, with my right hand . . . if another man came at him with a knife . . . that's me, too, the other man is my left hand and the ruler is the knife . . . if the first man could somehow turn the knife around and stick it into the second man, all while he's crouching down.'

Chris considered this wisely.

'Yes,' he said at last. 'I think he could.'

'Thinking isn't good enough. The first man could be sent to prison for a long time – so I have to be sure.'

'Did the first man kill the second man?'

'Well . . . yes.'

'Have you seen him?'

'The first man? No.'

'The second man.'

237

'Yes, Chris, I've seen him in the mortuary. I've examined his wounds and I know that the knife went into him at a certain angle, in a certain way. I'm trying to see if the first man could have done that when he was attacked while he was tying his shoelace.'

Chris nodded. I was not sure he really comprehended what I was saying. He just accepted that his father did some strange things.

'I came to show you my biology book. I got the highest mark of anyone.'

Of course! My son was here for a reason. And I had been so engrossed I had told him about my work without even asking what that reason was. We looked at the biology book together and I exclaimed with great parental pride over his run of As and eventually Chris left looking cheerful and I continued my experiment. Despite trying very hard, I simply could not contrive a way for a crouching individual to deflect or push a knife held by an assailant into the assailant's chest – not if the result was to be such a high, horizontal track into the pillow. I mean, body. As I had strongly suspected, this case was a straightforward (in both senses), standing stabbing injury.

There was a small knock at the study door.

'Daddy, we both think he did it,' said Anna, bursting in.

'Who did what?'

'Well, Chris was the first man, tying his shoelace and I was the second man, coming at him with a knife and –'

'You didn't use a real knife, did you?'

'No, I used my pen. Anyway, Chris easily turned it

round and stabbed me, so we think the first man is a murderer.'

'Right. Well. Thanks.'

'Shall we show you? Or if you like, you could be the first man and I'll be the second man, I'm better at this than Chris.'

I felt that Anna, who must only have been seven years old, should not really be helping me reconstruct a homicide. If she ever caught me with a knife she tended to regard it as a bit of a joke. She responded to the idea of dead bodies as something unsavoury but the full meaning of death was still lost on her and she had certainly not seen a body, not even a photograph. Not only were the children taught to knock on the study door, I always carefully hid any police pictures on a high shelf.

'Just what game are you playing with the children!' demanded Jen, appearing from the living room, her face thunderous.

'No games, Chris came in, so I told him what I was doing.'

Jen rolled her eyes.

'I leave my work at the hospital,' she said pointedly.

Chris and Anna eventually would understand fully what my job entailed but, for now anyway, they were told simply to inform anyone who asked that I was a doctor. They had picked up the fact that I was a specific sort of doctor, that I helped the police and that my name appeared in the newspapers, but they had no real idea what a forensic pathologist was. Although around about this time they began to realize that my speciality did not make people 'better'. In our household it was fairly normal for Dad to stick rulers and knives into pillows and pieces of meat and, so far, Chris and Anna seemed not to have realized that other people's fathers didn't do that.

Today, the defence team in that stabbing case by the canal might successfully offer a manslaughter plea of loss of self-control. A post-Savile jury might decide that seeing 'a red mist' because your friend was sexually imperilling your thirteen-year-old sister is enough of a trigger. There were plenty of statements from family members that confirmed how upset and furious the brother had been at her possible abuse by his friend.

For the modern defence of loss of self-control, it must be proved that a person of the defendant's age and sex with a reasonable degree of tolerance and self-restraint, would lose control in a similar way. I think the young man would have had a good chance of showing that. But for loss of control the defence must also prove that there was no premeditation. The pitfall for this defendant would be that the murder might have appeared premeditated if he had actually carried the knife to the canal that night. He had explained why his fingerprints were on the handle but he would have had to persuade the jury that the victim had been the one to take the knife from the kitchen before they went out for their walk.

This homicide happened long before the reforms of 2010, in less enlightened times. Loss of control was not a defence. There was then no hope for the young man who was so anxious to protect his sister. The charge was murder and he was found guilty: an open-and-shut case in the 1980s.

A routine murder, but one in which the precise angle and track of the stab wound provided important evidence. And it very often does. Not just the track, but, once the knife is in the body, its subsequent movement inside an organ can sometimes chart the respective movements of victim and perpetrator. As my casebook thickened, I became increasingly convinced that knife wounds could tell all, if only we could hear what they were saying. I wanted to compile a really comprehensive analysis of tracks, angles, hilt bruises . . . I was always rooting around in the kitchen at home for another knife to stick into another piece of meat. In fact, I bought so many knives of different shapes and hilts that, going home at night, had the police been in the habit of stopping and searching middle-class, white men, I could frequently have been arrested for carrying offensive weapons.

To the continued disgust of my family, I now used pork bellies or cow kidneys for my stabbing exercises. It was extremely hard to reproduce quite the feel of pushing through human skin, muscle and then an internal organ – perhaps because supermarket meat is seldom fresh. In reality, people who have killed with a knife are usually astonished by how easy it is. Once the blade has cut through the clothing and the skin, the inner body tissues put up little resistance. Only moderate force is required to penetrate major organs like the heart or the liver, and so even perpetrators with little strength can kill by stabbing. A lot of murderers say, 'I didn't mean to kill him!' What they are actually saying is, 'I didn't think that what I was doing would kill him.' And this is more likely to be true when knife murderers say it than others. Knives give the murderer an immense advantage over their victim even if the victim is much stronger. No wonder women so often turn to them.

And did I prove, after all these experiments, that it is possible to read the history of a murder by reading the stab wounds like a book as I had hoped? Well, no. But I did find knives could tell a lot about a homicide. I developed the ability to sketch a murder weapon with some accuracy, based on the track it had left in the body. And when the police offer me a series of possible murder weapons, I can exclude most and, if the right one is presented to me, generally pick it out.

Just eight months after the Clapham rail disaster I took a call early one Sunday morning to warn me that there had been another disaster. It was August and Iain was on holiday and I was the forensic pathologist in charge of London and the south-east of England. At this stage, no one knew how many bodies there would be but one thing was certain: there would be bodies.

This time catastrophe had occurred not on the railway but on the River Thames. I waited for more news before setting off and my first stop was the Police Pier in Wapping. A leisure boat had sunk somewhere near Southwark and bodies recovered from the vessel were here. That was all I knew.

An old police sergeant greeted me and to my astonishment he was close to tears.

'Almost got my thirty years in, Doc. And now there's twenty-five dead from the river, twenty-four on the boat, another one picked up this morning eight bridges upstream at Vauxhall. Never thought I'd see anything like this. They're all kids. Kids in their twenties.'

So the boat that went down must have been one of those party vessels, the sort people hire to cruise up and down the Thames. I had seen them and heard them many times. Young people on the deck, clothes fluttering under the lights like giant moths. Laughter and music discernible from either river bank. Through the windows, the shadows, colours and movement of a dance floor.

The sergeant added, 'Doc, the police surgeon's already been in and certified them all dead.' And now he really began to cry, walking away, shaking his head. I heard him blow his nose before opening the door and going back to the front desk to fend off the press.

Wapping Police Pier is a Victorian police station standing right beside the river. At the back, an area had been designated the temporary mortuary. It was just a room, really. Its concrete floor was nearly covered by body bags. All of them lay open and in each one lay the body of a young adult. All dressed for a party, many in bright colours. I looked across this devastating scene and I noticed something strange. Their clothing had been disturbed. Dresses were displaced, trousers opened . . .

I immediately went back out to the sergeant. He grimaced.

'Police surgeon opened all the clothes. Think he might have been checking what sex they were.'

I wasn't pleased but there wasn't much I could do about it now. Probably they had been overwhelmed by events and had needed to feel that he was doing something, anything, useful: check pulses, listen for heartbeats. I had seen this sort of reaction before – even highly trained professionals want to 'do something', when they know full well that the correct thing to do is absolutely nothing.

I then went to Westminster. I knew the deceased wouldn't stay long in the temporary police mortuary. I wanted to ensure that Westminster mortuary was prepared for the large number of bodies that was about to hit them.

Oh no. I remembered that the usual manager, Peter Bevan, was on holiday. His deputy was in charge and I had never found this man to be anywhere near as organized or efficient as his boss. Peter's calm, capable organizational skills were exactly what we needed when managing a mass disaster. However, at least the staff were busy preparing for the huge intake and all the post-mortem tables and necessary equipment were ready. The sight of these preparations gave me, for the first time, a sense of dread that was something close to nausea. It was fleeting. But powerful.

With another pathologist under my supervision, I agreed to return the next day when the bodies had been brought over from Wapping to start the examinations.

Gradually, the facts emerged. On that calm summer night, a huge dredger had collided on the Thames near Southwark Bridge with a small pleasure boat called the *Marchioness*.

The *Bowbelle* had dumped its cargo of gravel at Nine Elms and was proceeding back out to sea to dredge for more. The *Marchioness* had been hired to celebrate a birthday and an international crowd of young people was partying on board.

Initially, the *Bowbelle* hit the little *Marchioness* at the back on the starboard side. This caused the pleasure boat to rock and keel over: a witness said the *Bowbelle* then 'mounted it, pushing it under water like a toy boat'. In fact, the anchor of the dredger cut right through the pleasure boat's upper deck before a second impact pushed the back of the *Marchioness* round to starboard, causing her to roll over.

Here are some survivor statements:

I felt a jolt . . . then I noticed the stern moving out in a starboard direction . . . I saw water come through the open window. I felt the boat keel over . . . I remember turning around to head towards the windows to escape . . . as water started coming in . . . I knew the boat was going to go down. Within a matter of seconds, the lights went out. Everything was in darkness . . . I was then thrown forward by a wall of water. The whole boat filled instantly . . . When I surfaced I was some distance away from the *Marchioness*, which was partly submerged . . .

I . . . felt the right-hand side of the boat . . . dip down suddenly . . . As the boat tipped over, water came flooding in through those open windows on the right-hand side. Everybody who had been on the dance floor lost their footing and with me and chairs and everything moveable went sliding down to the right, down into the water which was filling the dance area incredibly fast. I went under water . . .

Suddenly the boat tilted onto its side and the toilet began to fill with water. I tried to unlock the door and get out. When I managed to get the door open the boat was completely submerged.

I felt the boat rock, then it all of a sudden sort of swerved round and I lost my balance. I think I fell against a table . . . I saw this hull coming through the boat, I saw this anchor coming in, glass started breaking, all the windows smashed and showered us with glass, water started pouring in . . .

A terrifying ordeal for the young people on board. All passengers' chances of escape were hampered by the great speed of the sudden rotation, loose furniture, darkness, the cold, turbid water and, for some, the lack of accessible emergency exits. The result was that, to get away, physical exertion and strength were required. Which compromised the survival chances of many.

A much later statement on the disaster made by Dr Howard Oakley, an expert on survival and thermal medicine, said, 'Sudden capsize is known to be a shocking experience, to which individual reactions would have varied from panic to calm determination to escape and survive . . . physiological responses to that shock are likely to have shortened the time for which victims could hold their breath, which would in turn have reduced the chances of successful escape.'

Within thirty seconds of impact, the *Marchioness* was lying at the bottom of the Thames. Fourteen vessels helped to rescue the living. But not for several hours, at least, were the dead retrieved. Many of the dead were probably trapped on the boat. Others must have been thrown overboard. The Thames is a treacherous river, deep and dark, with a rich mixture of currents and tides which are known to hide bodies for days and even weeks before giving them up. In fact, it was five hours before the first body from the *Marchioness* was found in the river. And almost two weeks until the Thames yielded the last one.

A drowned body – or a body which is immersed in water after dying some other way – will first develop opaque, wrinkly skin. Anyone who has spent too long in the bath will have an idea what this looks like. It is often called 'washerwoman's hands', the thick keratin layers on the fingers, the palms and the soles become macerated and the skin appears very white and wrinkled, whatever the ethnicity of the deceased. After a few days, if the body remains in the water, this macerated skin will begin to separate and it will, eventually, peel off.

I should also say, because it is relevant to what happened next, that the time it takes a body to float to the surface depends on the gas in the bloated and decomposing body. Generally, the obese surface fastest.

The *Marchioness* went down shortly before 2 a.m. on the morning of Sunday 20 August. By the end of that day, although I had, with a colleague from Guy's, viewed and organized the bodies, we still had no idea how many people on board had died. There were clearly a lot of survivors so we were harbouring hopes that there might be few further bodies.

By law, the coroner is in charge of those bodies and Westminster's coroner, Paul Knapman, came back to London from his holiday in Devon and met with me and senior police officers to agree how we would process the dead. As coroner, he had to establish positive identification of the bodies, and we discussed how he wanted to do this.

In mass disaster management, false identification is the biggest fear. This is obviously hideous for everyone, especially if a family later begins to suspect they may have buried the wrong body. The coroner rightly wanted the most secure and accurate identification methods that were possible. Now we have the option of DNA analysis but, although the subject of much pub discussion, DNA identification was just not available to us then. The two most secure means were still fingerprints and comparison of teeth with dental records.

The problem with dental records is that you, of course, have to know the name of the missing before you can begin to search for their dentist, and only when the name of the dentist is known can you request their records. And then that request can take a very long time to fulfil. This is especially true if records must come from other countries. And by now we knew that the partygoers on the *Marchioness* were a high-flying crowd from all over the world. That was clearly going to cause problems and delays.

As a result of all this, fingerprinting was the first choice of identifier. Fingerprinting plus dental records would be ideal. Absolute accuracy can be a time-consuming business, but the coroner took the view that accuracy was more important than speed. Which is surely correct, although I can understand this is very frustrating for anxious relatives.

Those who are trying to cope with the possibility of sudden bereavement after a mass disaster often cannot understand why the relatives are not simply invited into the mortuary to walk through the lines of fatalities to claim their loved one. Many relatives of the *Marchioness* victims, believing that identification must be easy, did in fact suggest that, if they could just be allowed into the mortuary, they could find their family member. I understand their need and their logic, but it is false. And it would have been utterly inhumane to allow this.

People find it hard to believe that, in mass disasters, visual identification is unreliable, especially so when death has been traumatic or the body has been immersed in water. But even the uninjured and undecomposed dead are often simply not recognizable to those who knew them as animated individuals. Without life, facial expression, movement, robbed of our essential selves, our bodies can look very different. And this is certainly the case when the dead have been held by the Thames for hours or days.

The fact is that relatives, even immediate family, when they are under great stress, are very likely to make mistakes. They may identify a body that isn't their relative. Or they may not correctly identify a body that really is their loved one. These are known as false positive or false negative identifications, and they happen more often than you might think. Later, perhaps much later, the identifying relatives sometimes worry they were wrong. And then change their minds. This can occur long after burial or cremation, when our ability to review the identification is lost. Add to the difficulties of identification the immense emotional trauma of having to look at many, many bodies in the mortuary to find the one you think may be your relative. With all my experience of death and dying I know I couldn't walk between rows of victims and reliably identify my own wife or child or parent.

I should say that being called on to see a body for identification purposes is quite different from seeing that body once police and pathologists are sure that the correct identification has taken place. I personally believe every relative who wishes to do so has an absolute right to see the body of their deceased. It is cruel to deny – for whatever reason – a family this chance to say goodbye personally. But the reality is that bodies may be injured, decomposed and smelly. We can do a lot with reconstruction, but we can't perform miracles. So it may take many hours of talking and discussing, of initially showing photographs of the body, before we can move into the room where the body lies. And then maybe more time again before the relatives will actually look at the body. Spending this time with families is crucial. So is care and compassion. We must do nothing to add to the trauma.

As unreliable as visual identification is the use of 'mobile' or moveable indicators, such as clothing, jewellery or wallets. These may be treated only as clues to identity because people swap jewellery or look after friends' wallets. And to use clothing, we would have needed to know exactly what the victims were wearing on the night of their death, relying on descriptions from others when such descriptions are seldom either accurate or available.

Despite this, the coroner was inclined to accept visual identification and mobile indicators – but only from those bodies recovered from the wreck of the *Marchioness* itself, and only as long as they showed no decomposition. In all other cases, the coroner instructed that mobile means of identification were not dependable.

The coroner's conclusion, when we discussed identification, was that fingerprinting of each body was essential. As a list of the suspected missing was compiled, police were despatched to homes (unless they happened already to have fingerprints on their database) to collect personal items on which fingerprints might be found, so that these could be used to match those taken in the mortuary.

Our problem was that these were drowned bodies. They were likely to be damaged, either by aquatic predators or by contact with rocks, bridges, boats or other underwater obstructions. Drowned bodies show all the discolouration and bloating of normal decomposition plus some much earlier skin changes. Even if retrieved from the water within a few hours, those inevitable 'washerwoman hands' can make fingerprinting difficult, and when there is a complete loss of the skin from the hands – elegantly called 'degloving' – well, then it can be extremely difficult or almost impossible to take fingerprints from the deeper layers of skin, the dermis.

At first this disaster seemed easier than Clapham because there was no severe mutilation of the bodies. As time went on, however, bodies arrived in worse and worse condition and decomposition became our nemesis.

Once again, each body travelled through a system. First, we described in detail clothes, jewellery and general appearance. I then helped remove the clothes and performed an external examination, describing tattoos, scars and anything unusual that might assist identification. Police officers made notes and the body was photographed and refrigerated.

The second phase was the full post-mortem, after which the internal organs would as usual be replaced in the body cavity and the body sewn up and made presentable for viewing by relatives.

Finally, I submitted a report about each of the deceased for the coroner, concluding with the cause of death: drowning. If he was satisfied with all this, especially the identification processes, he would open an inquest and release the body.

The first free-floating body was found in the Thames before 7 a.m. that Sunday morning. No more were found that day but in the afternoon the *Marchioness* was raised and when I reached Wapping police station, twenty-four had been found on board and arrived at Wapping in the warmth of an August day. They were tagged before being carried on to Westminster mortuary.

This mortuary is run by Westminster City Council. At that time, it had six holding fridges, refrigeration for sixty bodies and a further six units for extra-wide bodies. It had freezing facilities for eighteen bodies.

Whatever the outside temperature, bodies are refrigerated to a temperature of 4°C. This slows down the decomposition process but does not stop it completely. We do not freeze bodies until the post-mortem has been fully completed.

During a disaster, we work in a world of constantly changing information, often helping to revise and then re-revise it. The key problem for those managing the *Marchioness* victims was that no one had any idea exactly how many people had been on board the boat, nor who they were. So, within a couple of hours, while the rescue operation was still going on and before the first body had been found near Vauxhall Bridge, a telephone bureau had been opened to process information from friends and relatives that might help us identify victims. And by that afternoon, as Westminster mortuary prepared for its influx of dead, relatives of some on board had started to appear at police stations with photos of their loved ones and descriptions of what they might have been wearing.

By the end of that first day, the police believed that there had been 150 people on the *Marchioness*, of whom sixty-five, including those twenty-four bodies taken from the wreckage, were considered missing.

The next day I was back at the mortuary starting the long process of identification and post-mortem. We learned that eighty-seven survivors had identified themselves and we had twenty-five bodies, so we knew that if police estimates of the number of people on board were correct, there were a lot more bodies to come.

Expecting so many further arrivals, we worked as speedily as accuracy would allow. It was an extremely intense week. To see so many young people here was not just unusual, it was shocking. I was aware, as though in my peripheral vision, of the intense misery of parents fearing the worst, waiting for news. Bodies were laid out one at a time on the six tables in the post-mortem room and we worked our way doggedly from one to the next, feeling the greatest service we could perform for the bereaved was to do our job as efficiently as possible.

By eight o'clock that evening we had completed post-mortems on all twenty-five in the mortuary and, of these, thirteen had now been fully identified. The next day, Tuesday 22 August, we learned that the casualty bureau had received 4,725 calls from anxious relatives and had already amassed more than 2,000 documents on individuals believed to be on board. As we waited, a few more bodies were found in various places on the Thames, upstream and downstream of the disaster, and the police revised their estimate of the number of people on board the *Marchioness* down to 136.

By the end of the day there were thirty bodies in the mortuary and the police thought there were twenty-seven more to be found. But by now, immersion time in the Thames was taking its toll. Waterlogged skin was falling off fingers and the officers were having trouble getting prints using the standard inking process. The coroner called for dental records to help confirm the identity of the remaining fatalities but this would take time and relatives were anxious for news. So attempts to fingerprint continued but, as the hours went by, conventional fingerprinting was failing. It was now necessary to use a specialist technique and more sophisticated equipment. This equipment was based in a laboratory in Southwark – which had no facilities to manage bodies.

The routine process for individual bodies recovered from the Thames that could not be fingerprinted at the mortuary was to remove the hands, fingerprint them at the lab in Southwark, and then return the hands to the body. They were sewn back on to avoid distressing relatives, who, when the body is appropriately arranged, were unlikely even to see the stitches. The coroner allowed this and so the procedure was followed. Seventeen pairs of hands were removed.

That evening more bodies were found between Westminster and London Bridge, and then another, far downstream past Wapping. The next day, eight more bodies were found. One, retrieved at Cherry Garden pier on the south side of the river at Bermondsey, was wearing uniform and strongly suspected to be the *Marchioness*'s captain, Stephen Faldo. Another was nearby, then four more were found near HMS *Belfast*, not far from London Bridge. Two more were on the other side of the wreckage, upstream around Westminster.

That gave us a total of forty-four bodies. By now we had positively identified twenty-four of these. Of course, there was an assumption that every single body found on the river must be from the *Marchioness*, but this was unlikely to be the case: there are suicides and other deaths in the Thames almost weekly, and we had to be aware of this.

By the following day there were forty-eight bodies and, although we had been working as hard as we could, six were still waiting for post-mortems. The police were saying they now believed there had been 140 people on board the *Marchioness*: eighty-four survivors and fifty-six lost or missing. The dental records of all the known victims had been requested, those from abroad via the relevant embassies. That night, Wednesday, the casualty bureau closed, saying it had gathered all the information about the missing it could.

However, bodies were still being found and the police revised their estimates again. They thought there were eighty-three survivors and fifty-six lost or missing. But there was now a report, for the first time, of a fifty-four-year-old woman running the disco on the boat. This was followed by another report of a woman jumping into the Thames near HMS *Belfast* after a handbag full of bricks was found on the riverbank. As we carried out our post-mortems, some officers began to grumble at the way the casualty bureau had closed when so many inquiries were still outstanding. And by Thursday evening, there was a new development that pushed police estimates of the number of people on board up again: a group of gate-crashers at the party came forward to say they had survived the sinking – but a friend was missing.

Meanwhile, back at the mortuary, a request was sent to the lab for the return of the seventeen pairs of hands as soon as possible so that they could be reunited with their owners. Another eight pairs of hands were delivered to the lab.

There was not much more we could do now but wait. It was the Friday before the August bank holiday. Outside the mortuary, people were leaving hot London for the weekend. We were waiting for dental records to arrive, fingerprint information from the labs, or just more bodies: fifty had now been recovered. After all that frantic activity, the mortuary seemed almost eerily quiet.

No new bodies arrived in the mortuary over the long weekend. On the Wednesday, the police attempted to name the people still missing. One of them was the party's host, Antonio Vasconcellos, who had been celebrating his twenty-sixth birthday. Another was a Frenchman. And there was still one unidentified body in the mortuary, a man in his twenties: he may have been nothing to do with the *Marchioness*. Or he could be the gatecrasher, who had still not been named.

By the end of the week, forty-six of the fifty bodies in the mortuary had been positively identified and the others partially identified, meaning that we still needed more information to make it positive. Except for this one anonymous young man. Who was he? Nobody had any idea. He fitted no description.

Since he was carrying a distinctive key fob, the police photographed it and decided to release the picture to the press. So we had one person completely unidentified, and still two missing people: the Frenchman and Antonio Vasconcellos. We could stop worrying about the gate-crasher, though: he had shown up alive and well.

On Friday there was a major step forward in the identification of the mystery man. The distinctive key fob was taken to the Frenchman's flat and it opened the door there. Now only the party host was missing. That night the body of a young man was found downstream of the wreck, between London Bridge and Bermondsey, somewhere in that area broadly known as the Thames Upper Pool. We were fairly confident this was Antonio Vasconcellos, but after two weeks in the water we knew it would take some time to identify him positively. We were also confident that the other bodies in the mortuary were nothing to do with the *Marchioness* and the police were sure now that there were no more dead. The toll was fifty-one and there had been 137 people on board.

We had worked hard and, I felt, had served the victims and their families well. Only afterwards did I understand that, while I had been immersed in my work at the mortuary, a lot more was happening inside and outside it than I realized.

Everyone responds rapidly and wholeheartedly to an emergency. Everyone does their best at the time. So, although everyone, no matter how well meaning, should be held to account, it is hard to receive criticism afterwards for actions that may have been taken under extreme pressure in a crisis. The emergency and follow-up services, after many of the 1980s disasters I listed earlier, frequently found themselves on the receiving end of some very angry criticism. It is such anger that very often fuels reform. This is nowhere more true than after the sinking of the *Marchioness*.

I learned that, although some relatives early on identified their dead at a special viewing room at the mortuary, many others were told, due to late recovery of the body and the extent of the decomposition, they could not, they were not allowed to, see their loved ones. Sad reunions of the living and the dead do not usually take place at the mortuary: more often the body is moved to the undertaker's first. But undertakers, as well as the police, later claimed they had been told such viewings should be strongly discouraged and, even in the face of opposition, relatives should be refused access to the dead.

I do not know who ordered this or why. When I learned of it, I assumed it was the result of misplaced compassion, because someone thought that seeing a son or daughter in a state of decomposition is traumatic. However, that person clearly did not know that *not* seeing them is even worse.

One relative later wrote:

We were never actually prohibited from seeing [our daughter] but were talked out of doing so at every stage . . . when I went to the undertaker's expecting to

259

see her, the coffin was already sealed . . . I could not sit in a room with a box and so walked out of the funeral parlour. I feel very strongly that I should have had the opportunity of time alone with her. [Her mother] . . . has since seen photographs of [our daughter] and from the photographs there really is no reason why we should not have seen her.

Another wrote:

On Friday 25 August I was told by the coroner's officer that my son was not recognizable as a human being. On Thursday, 31 August, the undertaker phoned me to say they had collected [his body]. I went immediately to their premises and asked for the coffin to be opened. I wanted to make sure that I had found my son. The undertaker told me that he had been given orders not to let me view my son's body. This made me extremely upset. I was never given the opportunity to see him, to touch him and to say goodbye to him. The undertaker told me that he had been an undertaker for twenty-five years and he had never before been told that relatives could not view a body. 'I was told the coffin was sealed and it must be kept sealed,' he said. Since it is the undertakers who place a body in its coffin and they are the ones to close it, this was clearly untrue.

I still worry whether it is in fact my son who we buried. I think the root of this concern is that I was never allowed to see him . . . there is an additional concern that the bodies may have got mixed up . . . [Later] I looked at photos of his body. They were far less horrific than I had expected . . . I could not help feeling ill at ease with how things had been arranged . . . My concerns about whether I was ever given his body have meant that I have, in the past, sought an exhumation order.

I had no idea why the relatives of the *Marchioness* victims had been denied access to their loved ones: this seemed a cruel and unnecessary decision. It was to be a few more years before further information emerged to offer us – the relatives and those of us who had worked on the case – a possible reason why bodies were not seen and coffins not opened.

## 23

Early autumn, 1992. Jen was now a doctor. She had graduated the previous year and we had gone to her results night disco at the medical school bar, where I, at least, had felt rather geriatric. And then decided to enjoy the dancing. I was ridiculously proud of Jen but probably didn't show it. And maybe she was grateful to me for the support – the children, the house, the bills – but she didn't show that either. How hard it was to cross whatever chasm lay between us. It was much easier to ignore it, especially now that she was a junior doctor, working all hours, and I was so busy at Guy's.

Today, for once, I was working from home. Children at school, nanny off, Jen at the hospital. The daytime streets were quiet, much quieter than the office. The room was comfortably warm: a dog flopped on each of my feet. And the desk was littered with pictures of a homicide in which I was completely engrossed.

On top of the post-mortem pictures and a book of photographs of the victim's clothes were the scene-of-crime photos. I could not forget that rather grey July day. The urban wilderness of a large, south London park. A path heavy with tree shade, lightened by the trunks of silver birches. The POLICE DO NOT CROSS tape wound from tree to tree.

I saw something white in the grass, among the trees,

which, from a distance, you could mistake for a discarded handkerchief. As I neared the handkerchief, a detective on either side of me, it grew larger and became more dissonant with its surroundings until, by the time I arrived, the contrast screamed between this green place and the human body which lay, blanched, mostly naked, below shimmering birch leaves. A young woman. Curled defensively. Stabbed many times. Her lower body naked. Sexually assaulted.

I waited for the police photographers to finish their work before I took her temperature and a few early swabs for semen. I felt her for rigor mortis and found that only her jaw had set. Then I examined the scene, looking at places where the ground had been disturbed, the detectives pointing out the bloodstains on the grass, noting crushed leaves and broken branches where there were signs of a struggle. This all took many hours. The body was at last removed to the mortuary, where, watched by the same grave detectives, I performed the post-mortem. In the comfort of my study now, I remembered that long, long night. How it was dawn before every one of the forty-nine stab wounds had been measured and documented, each track traced through the internal organs it had penetrated.

I looked up. The clock ticked in the quiet house. I reached for the post-mortem report and reread the conclusion. No natural cause had contributed to the victim's death. She had died of multiple deep stab wounds inflicted by a knife or knives about 9cm long, about 1.5cm wide at the hilt. She had struggled and had been stabbed right through her left hand as she tried to defend herself. Once she was dead her assailant had not stopped stabbing her. And once she was dead he sexually assaulted her.

There was immense public horror at Rachel Nickell's brutal murder. She was a beautiful, twenty-three-year-old mother who had taken her toddler to Wimbledon Common for a walk. The nation's shock put pressure on the police to solve this crime, and solve it soon. So immense was this pressure that the Met stepped outside its usual box. Officers talked to forensic psychologists about profiling the killer. And they talked to me about reconstructing the case.

I had all but given up hope of playing my part in a police investigation – ever since my first careful recreation of a crime, that bedroom knife murder, was spurned by the case detective. And now, for once, the police had come to me and *asked* for a reconstruction. Specifically, they wanted me to piece together the likely sequence of events that day, based on the evidence present at the scene and at my post-mortem findings.

I had recently been inspired by a convention of American forensic pathologists I had attended. For a while now I'd felt that, as a profession, forensic pathology wasn't developing much: we all rushed around on our cases and discussed them in the pub, but that isn't the same as development, of ourselves or of our profession. I went to American conventions for a different perspective and recently I'd found just that when I had learned that American pathologists were now encouraged to be a bit more Simpson-ish by participating in the investigation.

So I read through my own very thick post-mortem report on Rachel Nickell. The wound details went on for pages. Three wounds, on the chest and back, which I had numbered 17, 41 and 42, stood out from the rest. They were the only superficial wounds in a victim who had been stabbed deeply over and over again. Could these have been the first?

There is a moment at the very beginning of the chain of events which leads to a homicide such as this when the perpetrator has to get close enough to his victim to gain control. We know that establishing control is a particularly important part of most sexual homicides. In such cases, we often find wounds that are not deep enough to injure but scary enough to make a victim comply with an assailant's demands: these are 'prodding wounds'. Were 17, 41 and 42 'prodding wounds'? There was just one on the deceased's back – number 17 – while the others were high at the front of her chest. I looked at them again. I wondered if she was first prodded in the back. And then, did she turn to face her assailant?

In the scene-of-crime pictures, the most significant bloodstains were easy to discern. They were not under trees but in a place where the summer grass was left long and full of seeds, like a meadow. This was about five metres from the place the body was discovered in the late afternoon by a shocked mother with a toddler, dog and pushchair.

There was a second, smaller area of staining, much closer to the body's final position: it was adjacent to the forked birch tree under which the dead woman was found. And, of course, there were bloodstains beneath the body. It was safe to assume that the initial assault had taken place at the bloodiest site, that the victim had been moved to the spot under the tree, and then pulled a metre into that final position nearby.

Looking at the endless list of wounds, it was hard to decide which came first, but the gaping neck wounds must have happened fairly early on as they would have produced the most blood. That would also explain why the victim apparently did not scream. Her neck had been attacked with force and the pain would have been extreme. If that didn't stop her screaming, then the resulting damage to the muscles around her larynx would have done so.

The pictures of Rachel Nickell's clothes told me another part of the story. Her T-shirt was wet with blood, of course. But her jeans, around and below the knee, were muddy at the front. And blood-spattered at the back. I was absolutely sure this could only be because she was kneeling early on in the assault, while the initial injuries to her neck were inflicted.

Of course, with such injuries she could not have remained kneeling. She must have fallen. It seemed likely she had fallen forward and that her assailant had now stabbed her back – eighteen times in all.

Whichever way she fell, but especially if she fell forwards, her neck would have bled profusely onto the ground. Is that why the killer moved her to the second area under the tree? Or did he do this because by now she had died? Or because he feared he could be seen too easily here on the grass?

The pictures showed less blood under the tree but the distribution was wider. That is probably an indication she was lying here supine. I checked the pictures of her body at post-mortem. Yes, leaf mould on her back. This must, indeed, have been where he stabbed her front. If she was not dead when he moved her, she must have died very soon after. Even so, he continued to stab her body. In particular, he stabbed the heart and liver post-mortem. They were penetrated, but the dead do not bleed.

Next, I noticed that the leaf mould on her back was also visible on her buttocks. So here, under the tree, he must have ripped off her jeans. And during or after this, her body was pulled over to be sexually assaulted in its final, compliant position.

Did he continue to stab her afterwards? Or did he run off at once?

'In my opinion, the minimum length of time needed to inflict all the injuries would be three minutes,' said my post-mortem report.

I knew that because, as usual, I had re-enacted the moves here at home. If the murder had taken only three minutes, it certainly must have been fast and furious. And it gave every appearance of a frenzied attack. Even the coroner himself used this expression and the newspapers had certainly not been able to resist it.

I had also spent hours analysing the knife wounds – some of which showed evidence of the weapon's square hilt on the skin because the blade had been plunged in up to its maximum depth. And for the first time I had a body part scanned. Magnetic resonance imaging showed the exact track of the knife wounds in the liver. All this information meant that, although the police had already presented me with a variety of possible knives, each time I had confidently told them that, no, the wounds proved this could not have been the murder weapon.

When I finished listing the sequence of last events in the life of Rachel Nickell, a young woman whose name is widely known for the saddest of reasons, I felt bone tired. World-weary. I looked at the clock. Almost time to pick up the children and walk the dogs.

I switched off the computer and listened to the faint groan it gives when extinguished. The dogs knew that sound and woke up simultaneously, yawning and stretching. They watched as I locked the photographs of the crime in my filing cabinet where no one, least of all a child, would stumble across them.

Creating a reconstruction that really might help the police to find that young woman's killer did bring me great satisfaction. I would very shortly be forty and this level of work represented the sort of contribution I had always believed it was possible for forensic pathologists to make to homicide investigations.

The dogs were wagging their tails, waiting to go. I did not move. I did not want to come back to the here and now from this engrossing work. Because there was something I had to do. Before dogs and children.

Reluctantly I picked up the phone and dialled one and then another in the list of numbers I had made from the Yellow Pages.

'Hello, am I talking to the undertaker?'

'Yes, sir, what can I do for you?'

My father was dying in a hospice in Devon. He had advanced cancer and was receiving terminal care. A couple of days ago I had said my sad farewells there, as court cases and other commitments dragged me back to London. My sister Helen had arrived to see him and then my brother Robert. I was making this call now, knowing that probably none of us would feel able to when the right time came.

The voice at the other end sounded confused.

'Sorry ... I must have misheard. Did you say your father isn't actually dead yet?'

'I'm afraid to say he soon will be, and I thought I'd organize things now.'

'I see.' Was that shock or disapproval? I felt embarrassed.

'I'm actually a forensic pathologist so I ... I work with death all the time and I'm aware of the ... the practicalities.'

'Ah.' My plea of mitigation had been accepted.

The formalities were therefore sorted out and, when the call came to say my father was dead, I was released from mundane details and could allow myself to grieve. Not to cry. Of course. But to feel the immense loss of my good-hearted and much-loved father. He had somehow shuffled through a long retirement in Devon with Joyce awkwardly by his side. My life had not in any way revolved around him, but he was a constant presence. I phoned every Sunday, he wrote every fortnight. Always there. Except now he wasn't. Something vast and unknowable seemed to gape at me. The immensity of death, which I always managed to evade in the course of my work, startled me by engulfing me now.

A day or so later I went to Devon and picked up the relevant forms from the hospice to take them to the registrar of births and deaths as instructed. The envelope said: *Confidential. Do Not Open.*

Naturally I ignored this. My life is spent dealing with

confidential details of the dead and these were my own father's. As I waited at the registrar's I opened the envelope and studied the contents without a qualm.

A cold hand snatched the envelope from mine.

'Just what do you think you're doing?'

'Well, I was reading the –'

'If you can read, you will have seen that these notes are confidential. You had absolutely no right to open them.'

My knuckles rapped, we proceeded to a small, shabby room for the formalities. Except that I had already seen on the paperwork that the doctor had given 'Carcinoma of prostate' as the cause of death. In the doctor's scribbled writing, it looked like 'Carcenoma of prostate'.

I watched as the registrar, still stony-faced, laboriously wrote the death certificate.

I said, 'Excuse me . . . carcinoma is actually spelled with an i not an e . . .'

She looked daggers at me.

'I . . . I'm a forensic pathologist. That's why I was interested to read my father's notes and . . . well, I write the word carcinoma all the time and I can assure you it is spelled with an i.'

The woman glared.

'The doctor has spelled it with an e. It is my job to write the cause of death exactly as it is given. Therefore, I shall write carcenoma because that is how the doctor has chosen to write it.'

So my father's death certificate, which I had to send out many times, each time with a shudder of deep irritation, gave him a new and entirely unknown cause of death, called carcenoma. It would have annoyed him as much as it annoyed me. Although he would have enjoyed his unique place in government statistics.

Two days before my mid-life birthday, the Shepherds gathered in Devon for a much bigger event. Our father's funeral. Here was Helen, who lived in the north of England with her family. Here was Robert, who lived in France with his wife. Despite the geography, we all remained close.

The night before the funeral, we had a family dinner with all the children but, I am sorry to say, without Joyce. I hope this wasn't unkind of us. I did remain in touch with her for the rest of her life and took responsibility to see that she was housed and cared for. But that night, we didn't want to censor any story about our father that predated her; we wanted to be free to exchange anecdotes about that wonderful man and his own special character. Not all of them were to his credit but all of them he would have endorsed and enjoyed. We laughed a lot and drank his health and it was truly an appreciation of his life.

To die greatly admired by your children is no mean feat. He had been the eldest child in a large family and when there was not enough money for education, and perhaps not enough love, to go round, he set out to create both those things for himself and his own family.

Immersed in a sense of loss, but also of harmony and support among Shepherds, we drove back to London, the kids in the back, me at the wheel, Jen at my side grabbing the opportunity for some sleep because junior doctors need all the shut-eye they can get. Another family, another generation.

In fact, I felt some reluctance to leave Devon and go back to work. Guy's was a busy, stimulating, friendly place and I loved my job. But, unfortunately, I'd run into turbulent waters lately. First, I was roundly attacked by my colleagues for complying with the police request for a reconstruction of Rachel Nickell's murder.

'You're stepping right outside your area of expertise,' they said.

I pointed out that, actually, I had relied entirely on my expertise for the reconstruction. 'And this is the way forensic pathology's definitely moving in America,' I added.

They were unimpressed by the way forensic pathology was moving in America. They shook their heads. They said, 'When they arrest someone, and the prosecution uses your reconstruction, defence counsel will slaughter you in the witness box.'

By now I'd experienced enough public humiliation as an expert witness to know this was probably true.

My other worry was the *Marchioness*.

That tragedy had occurred three years earlier, but somehow the wreck of the pleasure boat kept resurfacing. Of course, the grief of those who had lost someone in the disaster could never end – and right now their grief was turning to anger.

We professionals might have thought it was over for us: some parts of the rescue and its aftermath had not gone smoothly but the focus of attention since the collision had been on its causes. There were many safety systems that should have been in place on the Thames that night and weren't, and it was generally believed that the disaster happened because neither vessel saw the other in time – because neither kept a proper look-out. However, whatever the reason, the enormous *Bowbelle* had clearly ploughed into the little *Marchioness*, and criminal proceedings had followed against the *Bowbelle*'s master.

Victims' relatives were furious that the master had been drinking heavily the afternoon before the disaster as he waited for the tide to change so that the dredger could head downriver. But experts (who didn't believe that the old RAF rule of eight hours from bottle to throttle had a marine application) said the master had substantially slept off this alcohol intake in a nap before setting off that night. So the charge against him was his failure to keep a proper look-out.

The coroner was forced by the Director of Public Prosecutions to adjourn inquests into the deaths until this criminal trial was over – but there never really was a result. Two juries failed to reach a verdict on the culpability of the master of the *Bowbelle*, and a later attempt to prosecute the dredger's owners privately also faltered.

After the *Bowbelle* verdict, or lack of one, the coroner decided it was not in the public interest to reopen the inquests as by now there had been close examination of the causes of the collision and safety had greatly improved on the Thames. But his decision added to the relatives' pain: some believed this was biased thinking, particularly after he made some unguarded comments about one of them to the press, which were subsequently published. The relatives not only wanted a full inquest, they wanted a full public inquiry. Both requests had been stonewalled and it is to their great credit that their determination did not falter. They intended to pursue the possibility of an inquest through the Court of Appeal.

However, their anger was fuelled by their recent discovery – and unfortunately many of them made this discovery through the Sunday newspapers – that hands had been removed from some bodies in order to identify them. Even more upsetting than that, it had now been learned that the hands were sent back to the mortuary but, unforgivably, some were never actually returned to their bodies. And relatives suspected that the only reason they had been denied access to their loved ones before their funerals was not because the bodies were too decomposed for viewing but because they lacked hands.

Everyone now directed their anger at the pathologist in charge. That pathologist was me. In their position I, too, would have been angry. But it was wretched to become the focus of such fury. It was no use saying to heartbroken, bereaved people that hand removal was routine in these circumstances. It was no use explaining that fingerprinting the decomposing drowned invariably requires laboratory technology which cannot be carried out at the mortuary. And it was too late to ask whether, just because this removal was standard at the time, it really was an acceptable routine.

In fact, neither the decision to cut off the hands of some victims, nor their actual removal, nor the failure to replace them was anything to do with me. However, my denials were ignored and my protests taken as somehow incriminating. My photo (looking rather seedy, tie always flying behind me in a sinister fashion) kept appearing alongside newspaper articles, accusatory or snide in tone. I received phone calls from journalists at all hours of the day and night. I was frequently doorstepped. One hack appeared, as though by magic, in the office. I found him sitting by my desk with solemn face and an ominously open notebook.

As for my colleagues, their headshaking over my contribution to the Rachel Nickell case continued into my handling of the *Marchioness* case. They asked, couldn't I have stopped the hands from being removed? Especially as, in most cases, other forms of identity were rapidly available. After all, hadn't the police reported that they were being swamped with dental records from across the globe? So surely I should have intervened in the idiocy of the hand removal.

My colleagues did agree, however, that they were all speaking without any experience of a mass disaster, and certainly not one due to drowning. And they agreed they were speaking with the advantage of hindsight, admitting they themselves probably would not actually have intervened in what was police standard practice at the time – especially since it had been authorized by the coroner.

Iain, head of department, maintained a sphynx-like silence on the whole matter, as he did on any important cases which he was upset at missing. I felt entirely alone with the fury of the press and the *Marchioness* relatives, a difficult position, no matter how much I sympathized with that fury.

Pam, who might have offered me some support, was no longer our chief organizer. Quite late in life she had fallen in love with a widower and stepped into the role of wife and stepmother. She didn't even try to mix pathology with home-making. She recognized that the demands of running a family did not allow space for the complexities of the pathologist–homicide interface. We had bidden her a sad farewell, the other assistants then all reshuffled, a new junior appeared for us to introduce to our murky world of London murders and the capable Lorraine was put in charge.

Oh, and there was a new pathologist.

One day a tall, blonde, leggy woman had strolled into the office. She wore a short skirt and a friendly smile and had cheekbones which looked as if they had been cut out of stiff white paper with sharp scissors. The other staff barely had time to look up from their desks before Iain, as the most alpha in an office of alpha males, shot out of his seat and claimed her, yes, like a Neanderthal, because in the last century the male sex was a great deal less evolved.

Vesna Djurovic was a forensic pathologist, half Serb, half Croatian, from what was then Yugoslavia. She was the, in those days, unusual combination of breathtakingly glamorous and highly skilled. She had been practising in Belgrade and was now looking for a job in London. She not only found a job at Guy's but also something she had perhaps not expected: a husband. Iain was already married and the resulting manoeuvres were complex and difficult, but, in so far as our dark landscape of homicide could shine with a celebrity couple, Vesna and Iain were soon it.

Jen and I could never be such a couple. With Vesna and Iain in forensic pathology together there became more social events involving partners but we were too busy to join in most of them. Jen had just finished her house officer year. Her shifts were thirty-six hours, which meant long days and alternate nights in the hospital. However, this pattern was just beginning to ease now because she had started to train as a GP, at the same time finding what was to become her particular interest: dermatology.

I knew that, at this stage of her career, she needed a lot of support. I'd needed it too, and she'd been there for me. Now I was trying to do the same for her. Becoming a doctor was such an achievement when she hadn't even started studying until she was over thirty. Probably I didn't express my pride often enough. I hope I expressed it sometimes. I mean, at least once, for heaven's sake.

Now our paths seldom crossed, and when they did we often argued. There didn't seem to be a mechanism to help us find our way back to a safer, happier place. I knew some couples reconciled in a loving, kind way, but I had never seen it happen – certainly that kindness had been lacking in my father's relationship with my stepmother – and I wouldn't, or perhaps couldn't, play the game. How exasperated my good wife grew with her busy, distracted husband.

'Why won't you let me love you?' Jen would cry. 'Why are you so quiet all the time?'

We went for counselling. I agreed to it, but all the same I felt as if Jen was hauling me up before the beak.

'His mother died when he was nine,' she said significantly. And the counsellor nodded, also significantly it seemed to me. Were they old friends, these two women, or was all womankind in some kind of conspiracy?

'What would you like Dick to do for you, Jen?' the counsellor said.

'Just put his arms around me and tell me he loves me! That's not much to ask, is it?'

'And Dick? What would you like Jen to do for you?'

I thought. But not for long.

'Make me supper,' I said.

The counsellor leaned back in her chair, eyebrows raised.

Jen's lack of culinary skills had always been a bit of a joke.

'Preparing and giving me a meal. That would be an act of love. But I'm always too busy looking after everyone to receive and Jen's always too busy with her training to give.'

'So, Dick, you feel you look after everyone?'

'I'm not complaining. My father did it too, he brought me up. I'm pleased to care for the kids and cook and be there for them, that feels normal. It's just . . .'

My father had done all those things. But there had been his anger too. The way it occasionally just exploded out of him, whatever the collateral damage to those around. Now I began to wonder if that had in fact been the welling up of some great unhappiness. My father had been unhappy. Maybe I, too, was unhappy. It occurred to me for the first time that my marriage might be improved if, like him, I sometimes lost control and allowed my feelings to erupt. But, if I had any such feelings, they were firmly buried in some inaccessible place. And if I couldn't even cry, how could I erupt?

'Yes?' said the counsellor. I had forgotten that I was sitting in this room now in Clapham with ambulance sirens blaring outside and my wife and a counsellor watching me, waiting for me to speak.

She prompted, 'You do the cooking and a lot of child-care but it's just . . . what?'

'I'd like Jen to show me she loves me by doing things sometimes.'

The counselling didn't last long. Somehow it fizzled out, or maybe we were too busy. Our children were still primary-school age, they were happy and healthy and we worked hard to create a loving home. There was often noise, sometimes music, sometimes laughter. Jen and I were both fully involved in jobs we loved. We were comfortably off. I had joined the parents' choir at the kids' school and by now I had become a loud, shameless and, I fear, usually tuneless singer. Jen, Chris, Anna and I all sang our way up the motorway to holidays full of sand, rock pools, mountains and moors on the Isle of Man, where we were received by generous and cherishing hosts. Our lives were surely good enough.

## 24

My fortieth birthday coincided so closely with my father's death that it was inevitable I would start to contemplate my own demise. I did not fear death, but did not much like its predecessor, senescence, the preprogrammed process of ageing. By now I had seen so many bodies that I was all too familiar with the progress of senescence and had a good idea what some of my own vital organs must look like.

At forty, I knew that, on my lungs' smooth surfaces, tiny black dots were already forming into lines, making tree-like patterns. In their own way the patterns might be rather beautiful, but this was filth: the sooty pollution of London, which alone had probably ensured that I already had a degree of emphysema – even without the twenty or more cigarettes I smoked each day. I wasn't the only smoker, of course. My colleagues smoked, and we worked in a perpetual blue haze. At home, Jen smoked. On the Isle of Man, her parents smoked. Everywhere, our friends smoked. In 1992 we all smoked, we smoked in pubs and restaurants, we smoked on trains, at our desks and on the bus. We knew it was bad for us, we knew that cigarettes contained over 4,000 constituents, many of which are toxic, from hydrogen cyanide to cadmium to benzopyrene, but we put up with all that for just one ingredient: nicotine. So far, we'd been young enough to think we were invincible. Now I knew that I must stop smoking, and I might be rewarded with an extra ten years of life. Although the structure of my lungs must have been irreparably damaged, and inevitably that damage would increase over time.

Pumping blood through damaged lungs is hard work for the heart, and I hoped that the right side of my heart was not already enlarged by struggling with this extra burden. As for its left side, I knew that, if I couldn't learn to control my reaction to stress, then my blood pressure would rise and my left ventricle would thicken trying to cope. The heart is an organ one can hold neatly in the palm of one's hand. So small but so steady, a little fist, clenching and unclenching seventy times a minute, day and night, year after year, 30 billion times over a lifespan. A faithful friend. Until it stops. It was down to me to repay its fidelity by managing my diet, exercise, smoking and stress levels. Just as I knew I should give my liver a rest sometimes from alcohol if I wanted it to carry out its magical repair work on itself.

Good resolutions, all of them. And quickly forgotten. An occasional whisky and soda seemed a good way of relaxing and it was much easier to light another cigarette than waste time contemplating how much I wanted one but couldn't have one. Stress-relievers, both. And I see in retrospect that there was no question of my giving up that year or the next, because 1993 heralded a period of very significant cases.

In April I performed a routine post-mortem on a young black man from south London who had been stabbed. There were a lot of such knifings then and this death looked like many others. They often turned out to be gang or drugs related. Racial attacks at that time were not immediately suspected. The only information I was given was that the young man had been in a fight. There was nothing to indicate to a pathologist that this was an unusual case, nor that the patient's name would become so well known, nor that I would have to give evidence about his death so many times.

Stephen Lawrence was a bright, ambitious eighteen-year-old who in no way fitted wider public perceptions of black youth in 1993. Rightly or wrongly, his recognition as a keen student who had a professional future was vital to changing attitudes and prejudices. While simply waiting with a friend for a bus he was stabbed twice by a group of white youths, who, we later learned, were hurling racist comments. There was a superficial incision on his chin, one deep stab wound that had penetrated his lung and another deep wound on the shoulder. Bleeding profusely, he somehow managed to get up and run over a hundred metres with his friend before finally collapsing.

In the months that followed I was shown by the police a total of sixteen knives, of which seven were possible murder weapons. One of these looked particularly likely. In July I was asked to make a further statement and said that, in my opinion, Stephen had been standing when he was stabbed around the right collar bone but had probably begun to fall by the time the second stab wound was inflicted on his left shoulder. Despite some very careful thought, I wasn't able to say with full confidence whether his assailant was right- or left-handed. Choosing one over the other might have made me look clever but the evidence was really too flimsy to risk exonerating the perpetrator.

That was the extent of my involvement with the police's investigation into Stephen's death at that time. I was unaware of the indifference and racism that were hampering it. The Lawrence family, however, were not. They understood there were witnesses, evidence and indeed suspects. But no charges were made.

Four months later, I was called to observe a coronial post-mortem in north London on behalf of the police. The post-mortem was actually performed by another pathologist: it was my job to watch, take any relevant samples and possibly participate if invited to do so but, on the other pathologist's insistence, I just watched. It was fairly clear to me that the woman we were examining had died of the adverse cerebral consequences of asphyxiation but there might be other causes of death revealed by the experts who were invited to give their specialist opinions on some of the organs – specifically the brain and the heart.

The deceased had obviously been involved in a fierce struggle and then manhandled into a body belt – that abdominal belt with the handcuffs attached. She was covered in cuts and bruises and had been bound at the thighs and ankles as well as the waist. Had she, in fact, sustained a head injury also? The brain pathologist would answer that question for me.

This case also turned into a significant one. Joy Gardner was a forty-year-old Jamaican who lived with her five-year-old son. That she had outstayed her visa and was in the UK illegally is not in dispute. Her mother and a large number of relatives were here, offering support while she studied, and she did not want to return to Jamaica.

Early one morning and without warning, immigration officers arrived at her home to deport her. They were supported by police officers, perhaps because resistance was expected. And Joy Gardner did resist. She must have thought she was fighting them for her way of life. She perhaps did not guess that she was fighting for her life.

Unskilled, untrained and determined to carry out orders, the officers struggled to get her into a restraining belt while she fought them and bit them, watched by her young son. In response to her biting, they wound almost four metres of one-inch-wide adhesive surgical tape – Elastoplast – around her mouth and face. They mistakenly believed that by leaving her nose clear they were allowing her to breathe. This is a myth. Covering the mouth can kill. It is not just a question of being able to breathe – it's a question of being able to breathe enough. Especially if a struggle has caused stress and exertion and massively increased the body's need for oxygen. In these circumstances, an individual simply cannot take in the oxygen needed, which may be many times more than usual.

Gagging can cause vomiting and, with the mouth blocked, vomit obviously cannot escape. So it gets into the airways. And a gag can press against the tongue, pushing it to the back of the mouth and blocking the back of the nose. Secretions also accumulate in the mouth and throat, and this further inhibits the ability to get air into the lungs. Gagging a distressed woman who had been struggling hard for many minutes was all it took to bring about cardiac arrest.

Joy Gardner was not strangled. There was no traumatic head injury. She had not inhaled her own vomit. She was asphyxiated by the gag. However, an ambulance crew managed to resuscitate her. That is, they restarted her heart and then rushed her to hospital where she was placed on life support. Sadly, her brain had been so badly damaged by the prolonged lack of oxygen that she died four days later.

There was a breadth of involvement in this case – hospital, police, family – and consequently her body underwent so many post-mortems and so much tissue analysis that meetings about Joy Gardner sometimes felt like pathology conventions. Among the most important were the brain specialists, since it had been alleged by the first pathologist, whose post-mortem I had watched, that she had died from a head injury. Finally, overall, there was broad, general agreement that she had died from asphyxia caused by the gag.

I wrote a detailed report examining all the possible causes of death, which, as usual, went through various drafts and revisions. In the meantime, there was a growing outcry from human-rights organizations and others. It seemed to many, especially members of the black community, that police officers who regarded deportation as a job to be done at any cost and that they had killed Joy Gardner by thoughtlessly over-restraining her.

You might remember that the first death in custody I encountered caused by restraint had left me feeling some discomfort at the coroner's verdict. That patient had both pneumonia and sickle-cell trait and so was deemed to have died of natural causes aggravated by lack of care. From that day, I had been concerned about the methods sometimes used by enforcers of the law: it was obvious that some simply didn't know how to restrain people safely.

And restraint – indeed, death from restraint – was definitely on the increase. Joy Gardner was restrained so that she could be deported. Other deaths were caused when the police tried to apprehend suspects, particularly if those suspects had sickle-cell trait. But most deaths we were seeing caused by restraint now were due to another factor: the spiralling use of just one drug. That drug was, of course, cocaine.

Cocaine blocks the brain's uptake of neural transmitters and the blockage can give continual, pleasurable stimulation: it gives confidence, euphoria and energy. Cocaine users can talk for hours, have heightened responses to physical stimuli, so sex is more enjoyable, and they have little need for food or drink. It can, however, lead to a greatly stimulated heart rate, agitation and psychosis. So, if restraint is required for a cocaine user, it is usually because he appears to be suffering from uncontrolled psychosis.

My first cocaine death came at about this time, and it was an early marker in Britain's rising cocaine use. A very large and muscular drug dealer (who was also himself an addict) was arrested, having just bought a large quantity of cocaine, and at once began to punch the two police officers detaining him. An officer stuck an arm around his neck but that was just one manoeuvre in what was pretty much a fight. The fight ended with the dealer's death. But how had he actually died?

A highly regarded neuropathologist confirmed that the dealer did not sustain a head injury in the fight, so that was not a cause of death. He may have been asphyxiated by the arm around his neck, but he showed only one of the three classic signs of this: insufficient to give asphyxiation as a cause of death. He had consumed a lot of cocaine, but his blood sample put him below the fatal level, so he probably did not die of an overdose.

Finally, I gave a combination of causes: the stress on his heart generated by his fight with the police, coupled with the fundamental stress caused by his cocaine use. Although a young man, he suffered from an inflammation of the heart muscle. Now this is recognized in cocaine users and sometimes called 'cocaine myocarditis'.

Charges against the two police officers were later dropped. But this was another case that left me with a sense of discomfort I could not ignore. There were simply too many deaths when police officers restrained people. They surely believed that they were simply doing their duty, and they certainly had no intention of killing anyone. But people were dying. I knew I would have to do something, but it wasn't clear to me yet what I could do.

While we waited to see if anyone would be arrested for Joy Gardner's death, headlines everywhere announced an arrest for Rachel Nickell's murder. It came as no surprise to me. I had been aware of the police's suspicions about a man called Colin Stagg. I knew that, in the absence of forensic evidence, they had set up a honey trap on the advice of a psychological profiler. They recorded intimate sexual conversations between Stagg and an undercover policewoman, hoping Stagg would reveal himself as Nickell's murderer. He did not, but the Crown Prosecution

Service thought that what he did say was incriminating enough. I answered a number of questions about the murder from the team targeting Colin Stagg and my reconstruction of events that day on Wimbledon Common was used as evidence for the prosecution. I was expected to appear as a witness at the trial the following year.

With Britain's most notorious murderer now believed to be safely on remand and awaiting trial, I was surprised to be called, in the autumn, to the body of another young woman. She had been the victim of an even more deranged attack than that on Rachel Nickell.

Jack the Ripper, who killed at least five women in East London in 1888, is still the stuff of film, fable and countless guided walks daily around Whitechapel. I suspect that the public is so fascinated by his gruesome crimes because they happened long ago. Samantha Bisset's name, and that of her killer, are barely known, I believe because she was the victim of such a truly shocking Ripper-type murder that the press, for once, was reluctant to inflict on readers the horrific information unfiltered by time's lens. I feel the same reluctance and do not here give details of this homicide.

Not only was Samantha killed and sexually assaulted, but also her four-year-old daughter. Whose body was then tucked into bed with her toys so that the first police officers on the scene harboured hopes, soon dashed, that she had safely slept through the murder of her mother.

I was called in by the coroner, my interest in knife crime now widely acknowledged, to carry out the second post-mortem on the bodies of Samantha Bisset and her daughter. This second post-mortem was not for the defence, since no one had been charged with the murder, but for the coroner so that the bodies could be released.

It had fallen to a colleague to visit Samantha Bisset's flat, where these crimes had taken place. Therefore I saw the scene only through the photographer's lens. I could imagine the terrible silence, how the usual camaraderie, the exchange of pleasantries, inquiries about families or holidays, the workaday stuff we use to remind ourselves of normal life when we are confronted by a homicide, how even that must have been impossible for all investigators in the home where these acts of cruelty and mutilation had occurred.

As I carried out the post-mortem, it became clear to me that the killer had been, like Jack the Ripper, something of a trophy-hunter.

I said to the police officers attending, 'If I didn't already know you've got Colin Stagg, I could really think this was carried out by the same bloke as Nickell's murder.'

The senior officer shrugged.

'No way; we've got Stagg and he's as good as confessed.'

'It's not that similar,' pointed out his colleague. 'No one mutilated Rachel Nickell.'

'Maybe he would have done if he hadn't run out of time. Maybe he wanted to enjoy himself killing her but he was in a public place and he just couldn't do that without getting caught. Killing a woman slowly in her own home probably would have been the next step for him, too.'

'Yeah, well, he's inside and he's staying there for the rest of his life,' said the officer. And soon the same could be said of the man who killed Samantha Bisset. Robert Napper was a twenty-eight-year-old warehouseman with a history of violence and mental illness. He had often been brought to police attention but somehow, perhaps due to poor record-keeping in those days before the widespread use of computers, he had always slipped under the radar. Now his fingerprints in Samantha Bisset's flat connected him to this crime.

On his arrest, the police were confident that they had taken two ruthless murderers, Stagg and Napper, off the streets. So it was a very great shock when, in September 1994, Colin Stagg was acquitted.

The case was thrown out by a judge who said that the police operation was nothing more than entrapment and that, because Stagg had been lured into talking to the undercover policewoman, anything he said was inadmissible evidence. I was as astonished as everyone else: the police had worked with many professionals on the case and it had not occurred to me to challenge their absolute certainty that Colin Stagg had killed Rachel Nickell.

Colin Stagg was released – but into a different sort of jail. He only had to walk outside his front door to be subjected to immense cruelty. The police, press and, most of all, the public, were still convinced that Stagg had murdered Rachel Nickell and somehow got off on a legal technicality. This belief was so widespread that it didn't even occur to me to draw attention once again to the similarity between Nickell's killer and Bisset's. I had learned only too well that expert opinion is marginalized by the system and, despite my brief foray into crime reconstruction, I was now firmly back in my box.

## 25

The relatives of those who died when the *Marchioness* went down had doggedly been pursuing their case all these years. Now they won a victory. When their attempts to persuade the coroner to reopen an inquest had got nowhere, they had turned to the Court of Appeal, which agreed that, by refusing them an inquest, the coroner was 'in real danger' of showing unfair, though unconscious, bias. As a result, an inquest was finally held by another coroner. Six years after the disaster, in 1995, the inquest jury agreed nine to one that the victims were 'unlawfully killed'.

There was no one to prosecute now, since two attempted prosecutions of the *Bowbelle*'s master had failed, but the verdict fuelled the relatives' belief that there should be a public inquiry. An action group continued to push for one. Their efforts were resisted by the authorities because there had been a complete overhaul of river safety as a result of the accident and it was argued that there would be nothing now to be gained by a public inquiry. The action group did not agree. Although it must have taken a great personal toll on them to continue their fight, the relatives insisted there was more to learn from their suffering and that a public inquiry was the best forum.

No one ever forgot the missing hands of the victims, and I was still held responsible for this. So, while I agreed with the reason the relatives wanted an inquiry, I dreaded it. Because the whole subject, including those hands, would surface yet again.

Pressure from the ground up on intransigent authorities was also evident in other important cases at that time. The investigations into the deaths of Joy Gardner and Stephen Lawrence, two years on, just seemed to be fizzling out. Except that there were many people who were not going to let that happen. First relatives, then whole communities, set out to mobilize public opinion by showing that, in the case of Stephen Lawrence, racism in the Metropolitan Police was hindering the investigation. In the case of Joy Gardner, they had to show that someone other than a court had decided to exonerate the officers involved.

At first, not much changed in the Lawrence investigation. However, to the astonishment of the Met, who insisted their staff had only been doing their job, prosecutors now charged three officers with the manslaughter of Joy Gardner.

At that trial, the QC gave me a cross-examination I shall never forget. Someone had leaked a copy of an early draft of my report on the case, and he pointed out that in my final draft there were over seventy changes. He dragged me through them, one by one, asking me to justify every word change, deleted comma or additional semi-colon. I felt my minor revisions (for instance, changing probably to possibly, or quickly to rapidly) made little difference to the overall case, but it was useless to say that in each draft I was refining and clarifying. The QC's clear implication was that I worked closely with the police and had been leaned on to make them appear less culpable for Gardner's death.

Our exchanges went something like this (and I am writing from memory since no transcript seems to have survived):

QC: Let us look at page 36 . . . why did you revise the word 'severe' to 'moderate', Dr Shepherd? For that was certainly a dramatic revision.

ME: It seemed on reflection a more appropriate description.

QC: But why was it more appropriate?

ME: Well, I considered all the facts again very carefully and revised my opinion.

QC: Are you sure that revision wasn't based on the receipt of further information?

ME: It was based entirely on my analysis of the case.

QC: But why would you make so extreme a change if you had no new information?

ME: I felt it was more correct.

QC: So . . . are you saying you . . . *changed your mind*?

ME: Indeed, I changed my mind.

QC: You simply changed your mind! Changed it on a, on a, on a mere *whim*?

I can see why he was suspicious. Of course, I regularly worked with police officers and it might have seemed a fair assumption that I was trying to please them. In fact, no one had leaned on me. Nor do I try to please. Yes, it might have felt awkward working with the Met if I had been instrumental in convicting three of its officers, that is the sort of dilemma I had always known a forensic pathologist must face occasionally. I had hoped that I would respond bravely to pressure and treat truth as my greatest ally.

Scandalously to many, all three officers were acquitted.

Personally, although I could not condone their actions, it was clear to me that the officers were, themselves, victims in a way: victims of an entirely flawed system. They had not been trained or informed how to restrain safely, they had not been warned about the possibly dangerous effects of their actions. They did not know the rights or wrongs of Joy Gardner's deportation. It was their duty physically to carry out the orders of bureaucrats who made their decisions on behalf of the British people. They thought that by restraining Joy Gardner they were simply doing the unpleasant job they were paid for. The fact that they did it so badly, I felt, reflected on their employer's bad practice.

Joy Gardner's sad death was a catalyst for change. For me it was the last straw. I knew now what I had to do. I became an active and enthusiastic part of, indeed sometimes the instigator of, bodies set up not just to review restraint procedures but to train properly anyone whose job requires them to restrain: principally police, prison and immigration officers.

It is impossible to know what will later be the significance, if anything, of one's own life: I'd like to think that in my case it will be my contribution to this change. It has largely been a question of making a nuisance of myself, running training courses, organizing conferences, writing reports, sitting on committees but, most of all, education.

Detractors of the police may be surprised that I found most officers extremely keen to learn correct and humane restraint: they, more than anyone, were aware of the deficiencies in their practice. They, more than anyone, knew that it wasn't just the families and friends of the victims who suffered, it was also officers' lives and careers which could be completely changed by the events of a few minutes. However, it was many years before every single organization which can lawfully restrain, from the Border Agency to the Youth Justice Board, finally endorsed the set of principles for safer restraint that we succeeded in introducing to Metropolitan Police training after the Joy Gardner case.

I became a member of the Independent Advisory Panel to the Ministerial Board on Deaths in Custody. It is jointly sponsored by the Departments of Health and Justice, as well as the Home Office. Sounds bogged down in bureaucracy? It isn't. That's just how much elbow power we needed to ensure the set of guidelines I wrote would be approved and adhered to.

The guidelines recognize that restraint can have a significant psychological effect on everyone involved, including those who witness it. They set out the principle that restraint should be used only when it is necessary, justifiable and proportionate to the perceived threat. And they acknowledge the possibility that poorly applied restraint can lead to death. So only approved techniques should be used, and only by trained, authorized staff.

Once an incident is underway, management is essential. I like to think that the guidelines here were influenced by my flying experience. Where there are two pilots in a plane, only one is in full control and, when control is passed from one to another, both pilots must verbally acknowledge this.

PILOT 1: I have control.

PILOT 2: You have control.

This routine brings clarity in a crisis. So I had the idea of transferring aviation practice to the crisis which is a restraint situation. In this crisis, the person who is responsible for the detainee's head, neck and breathing is the person in control. It doesn't matter if it's the lowest-ranking officer present, that person must take control by saying, 'I now have control of this incident.' The others must acknowledge with, 'You now have control of this incident.' Crucially, control gives the authority to order an immediate release and be obeyed.

There is more detail of course, involving medical monitoring, filming, records and debriefing. But the overall aim was to turn the rugby scrum of forcible detention into something used only when necessary, and in a well-managed and safe way. The result, I believe, has been a dramatic reduction in the number of restraint deaths by the authorities. In fact, it is now much more dangerous to be arrested by a fellow citizen or shop or nightclub security staff.

After the acquittal of the officers in the Joy Gardner case, there were calls for a public inquiry. Which were resolutely resisted. As for the Stephen Lawrence case, it was clear the police investigating knew some names and had suspicions. However, no prosecution followed and so Stephen's parents and friends began a heroic and dignified struggle for justice. They pressed ahead with their own civil prosecution of three of the five alleged killers.

I was called as a witness at this trial. Michael Mansfield QC was acting for the family in the unaccustomed position of private prosecutor. But it was all to no avail. The world watched as the proceedings collapsed almost before they started for lack of evidence considered admissible by the judge. Worse, the double jeopardy law at that time meant that the three who were tried could never again be tried for the same crime and it seemed that all possibility of justice was lost for the Lawrence family.

However, they did not accept this. They now demanded an inquest. It seemed public opinion was fully behind them. Many had been shocked by the acquittal of the officers involved in the Joy Gardner case. Now people were beginning to believe that the investigation into Stephen's case was hampered by the same sort of racism that had led to his death, and even a public inquiry – established only at the behest of a government minister and something considerably larger in scale and much more legally powerful than a coroner's inquest – began to look like a real possibility.

The Lawrence family's patience and persistence finally did lead to an inquest. The five suspects were ordered to appear. They did so, but refused, as was their legal right at an inquest, to answer any questions. The coroner, who is not legally allowed to actually name murderers, was helpless in the face of their rude silence. However, the jury found a way around that and cleverly concluded, in February 1997, that Stephen Lawrence had been 'unlawfully killed in a completely unprovoked racist attack by five white youths'. They might as well have said '. . . by the five white youths sitting over there'. And the *Daily Mail* more or less did so, publishing pictures of the five, naming them, and inviting them to sue if the *Mail* was wrong.

Public scorn at the failure to apprehend Stephen's attackers reached such a pitch that at last it really began to seem that demands for a public inquiry into the Met's investigative failures would be met. I was personally delighted by this strong move for change which was now forcing a rethink in official and police culture. It had not escaped my notice that so many of the deaths in custody or under restraint I had been dealing with were the deaths of black people, and, put simply, the potentially increased vulnerability of some individuals through sickle-cell trait certainly did not explain this disparity. I could see change was necessary, but I could not imagine how change might come about. It never occurred to me when I examined the body of Stephen Lawrence that precisely those knife wounds would, over the next twenty years, be the precipitating factor in that change.

## 26

After about eight years at Guy's, I had itchy feet. The wing of Iain West had become more smothering than sheltering and, despite our friendship and his many promises to promote me, he had not done so. I applied directly to the medical school dean behind his back for a senior lectureship and was immediately promoted. But Iain really didn't want me or perhaps anyone else to become his deputy. As for his possible early retirement to embrace fully his country-squire lifestyle of huntin', shootin' and fishin', well, Iain made it clear that was not even on a distant horizon.

I looked quietly for other openings and continued with my work. By now, approaching the mid-1990s, both my children were at secondary school and occasionally I could glimpse in their young faces the adults they would become rather than the small children they had once been. It had always been hard to carry out post-mortems on children who were the same age as my own kids: this was probably the one time my hand wavered – momentarily – over a body. And now that they were growing up, there seemed to be more cases involving children. Had I been avoiding them before? Or were they really on the rise?

One day I was called to examine a baby who had died in his mother's arms at ten months. I found him to be well nourished and well grown. There had obviously been resuscitation attempts but there were no other marks on him, and certainly no sign of violence or trauma. The internal examination was just as unrevealing: there was not one indication of abnormality.

I waited for the toxicology, virus and bacteria test results but decided that if they were all clear I would have to give sudden infant death syndrome as the cause of death. The police were not too happy that I was thinking SIDS and promptly handed me a bundle of background notes. Ah. Now the case had a context, and what I read seemed to change things.

Officers had arrived at the mother's flat in response to her 999 call. She was twenty-two years old and lived alone after receiving death threats from the baby's father. Those threats – but also the mother's drinking habit – had placed the ten-month-old baby on the at-risk register. To protect them against the father, an attack alarm had been installed in the home.

When the mother phoned the emergency services at about 9 p.m. she sounded drunk and referred to a 'death in the family'. The attack alarm rang too, but only as police were actually on their way to the flat.

The police were concerned because, only a month before, this young mother had been convicted for being drunk in charge of her child. This is an offence that carries a fine and rarely a custodial sentence: its main purpose seems to be either to humiliate mothers into sobriety or to alert social services to the possibility of neglect or abuse.

On arrival, only seven minutes after her call, the police rang the bell. No one came to the door. They peered through the letterbox and could see the mother pacing up and down the hallway with the baby in her arms.

She was not panicking and there was no obvious threat, so they did not break in. They gently persuaded her to open the door, although she had great trouble doing this because she was so drunk. When eventually the police were able to enter, they found that the baby she had been cradling was dead.

All attempts were made at resuscitation. The mother was angry, aggressive and, of course, upset. A couple of hours later a blood sample was finally taken, and from this it was possible to extrapolate her blood alcohol level at the assumed time of the baby's death: that is, when she dialled 999. The level was 255mg/100ml of blood. It is illegal to drive above 80mg in England and Wales (now 50mg in Scotland) and for a less hardened drinker 255mg/100ml could possibly be a fatal dose. So we can conclude that, although she was clearly accustomed to alcohol, the mother was very drunk indeed.

The sample revealed no evidence of any drug use. However, she was too drunk to explain whether the child had died in her arms or in his cot or on the sofa or her bed. And she was unable to say where she had been at the time.

Perhaps your sympathy for the bereaved parent is now strained. Perhaps mine was. I had the baby's blood tested for alcohol and drugs. By now we had begun to recognize that some parents who drink or take drugs, in order to keep their children quiet while they do so, administer to them the same substances they enjoy. And sometimes they administer a fatal dose. However, when the toxicology report came, it revealed that this was not the cause of the baby's death.

There are fads in illnesses, as in most things. Their popularity waxes and wanes according to our perceptions. Sudden infant death syndrome, where an apparently healthy baby dies for no evident reason, gradually entered the public consciousness during the 1970s and 1980s and by the early 1990s it had become statistically significant, peaking at two per thousand live births.

SIDS was a welcome diagnosis for many pathologists. It seemed to explain the unexplainable and it cleared parents or carers of any blame. SIDS says that the baby did not die of any unnatural cause and so the assumption must be that it died of natural causes. But SIDS was not universally acceptable – there were some police officers and non-medical coroners who were sceptical.

In this case, the police suspected that the drunken mother's hand had been involved in the baby's death. This was reasonable in the circumstances, except that there was simply no evidence at all to support it. Therefore, having excluded all other possible causes of death, I was left with SIDS. There were many changes in my life immediately after this. And I was to look back on the cause of death I gave in that case just one year later and feel some surprise.

This was, in fact, my last case at Guy's. I had learned of the forthcoming retirement of Dr Rufus Crompton from my alma mater, St George's Hospital in Tooting. He was my former teacher and mentor, who now headed a department of which he was the sole member of staff. The opportunity to replace him was really exciting. St George's was willing to grow the department and if I got the job I'd be able to expand it along the managerial lines that I was always suggesting to Iain and which he completely ignored.

One grey day I asked Lorraine if Iain was free and then walked rather nervously into his office. It was a large room, filled with utmost chaos. Stacks of files and other papers teetered on the desk, on every shelf, on the floor and on the huge table at the centre of the room, which was used for meetings. When one was scheduled, Lorraine would move all the piles of paper off the table, finding some corner of the floor for them, and take away the overflowing ashtrays and the old cigarette packets. When the meeting was over, it would all start again. Judging from the clutter on its surface, I estimated that it had probably been over a week since the last meeting.

Iain was sitting at his desk and did not immediately turn his huge jowls towards me when I came in. This was perhaps not the best time to approach him, because I knew he was tired. Yesterday he had been shouting, which always meant that, whoever he appeared to be angry with, he was actually angry with himself, generally because he had failed to do something. Although of course he blamed Lorraine: she had not reminded him to produce that report on time. The report had almost certainly been sucked into the vortex of other files on his office floor but the court had been unsympathetic and ordered him to produce it by this morning at the latest. So he and Lorraine had been in the office until late last night, he dictating, she abandoning her shorthand pad and typing directly into the computer.

Now he sat with a menthol cigarette between his fingers. Another, forgotten, burned in the ashtray by his microscope. And a third lay, smoke spiralling from it, to one side of the room next to the flickering screen of his huge desktop computer.

I said, 'Iain, you've probably heard that Rufus Crompton is retiring . . .'

He raised his eyebrows. It had long been understood between Rufus, me and Iain that one day I might like to go back to St George's.

'I'm planning to apply for the vacancy,' I said.

He lit another cigarette from the end of the one he was finishing, looked around for an ashtray, or anyway one that wasn't already full, failed to find such a thing, and stubbed out the spent cigarette on the packet.

'I suppose you'll be needing a reference,' he said.

He smoked even more furiously than usual but did not betray emotion in any other way. He was cordial and wished me luck in my application and we agreed that, if we were both to run departments, we would not be rivals but highly co-operative with each other. I'm not sure either of us meant it, though. We were rivals already and now that we were to be equals in different hospitals that rivalry was unlikely to cease.

Leaving busy Guy's with its famous departmental head and plethora of fascinating cases to leap into the unknown was scary. I took a break that summer from post-mortems as I moved to St George's and began to set up the new department. It was essential for the police to recognize us and call us out, so, tedious though it was, I had to create a sound management and financial structure.

After a few months of this, I was surprised to find myself missing the mortuary, where I could use the skills I'd honed over so many years. When a pathologist friend on the south coast went on holiday I agreed to fill in for his routine coronial post-mortems. It was the school summer holidays. Anna and Chris were teenagers now. Anna was still at school but Chris had just finished his GCSEs and was hanging around at home, so I offered to take him with me. If he waited while I did a few quick routine post-mortems for the coroner – no homicides here, just sudden, natural deaths which required an explanation – then afterwards we could go for a walk along the clifftops. Chris was a relaxed sort of boy who was up for anything, so he was happy to sit reading in the car while I went into the mortuary to work.

I put on my kit. The mortuary staff had lined the bodies up on tables and prepared them for me: in those days that meant the bodies were still opened up, with the ribcages removed, and skulls opened too.

There was the usual small talk with the coroner's officer, during which I happened to mention that my son was waiting for me, reading in the car.

The coroner's officer clearly saw this as borderline neglect.

'I'll bring him to the office, he'll be more comfortable in there,' he offered. 'He can have a cup of tea.'

I was busy over an open body, PM40 in hand, when in the corner of my eye I saw Chris. He was walking through the post-mortem room with the coroner's officer. He seemed unperturbed. I, however, was extremely perturbed. I wanted to shout, 'Get him out of here!'

But I knew that would make the mortuary seem even more shocking for an unprepared teenager so, with a supreme effort of will, I winked at him from behind my mask and waved my PM40 jauntily. To tell the truth, I felt unmasked. All these years I had shielded my children from the reality of my work, without actually lying to them or misleading them, and now Chris had been unexpectedly exposed to it.

As we walked along the clifftops afterwards, there was a sort of mumbling between father and son.

'Er . . . were you all right with what you saw at the mortuary?'

'Didn't really bother me,' he said. 'But the coroner's officer was an idiot.'

Whatever subject they'd differed over (football, I think), it was more memorable for Chris than the sights and sounds of a working post-mortem room. He and Anna had sometimes actually come to the mortuary with me when I was working, so they were familiar with the smells and the clangs and the general ethos of the place. If the bereavement room was empty they would sprawl over the chairs doing their homework beneath the fish tank while beaming staff plied them with tea and biscuits. They had never actually asked what I was doing there, out of sight.

I did hope, without voicing this, that Chris wouldn't breathe a word at home about his expedition through the post-mortem room. And so, of course, he told Anna.

'Can I come to a post-mortem?' she demanded. 'It's not fair if Chris has been and I haven't.'

'I wouldn't exactly call that coming to a post-mortem . . .' I said.

And by now Jen had overheard.

'You saw *what*?' she asked Chris, throwing me an accusatory look.

'I'll have to get used to that sort of thing if I'm going to be a vet,' said Chris bravely. 'I'll have to cut up dead things all the time.'

'Well, I'm going to be a vet too,' said Anna. 'Or a doctor.'

Ours was a medical household and incidents and cases were routinely discussed, often quite candidly, although I still hid the case photos. If asked what their parents did, the children still answered, 'They're doctors.' If pushed, they would say, 'Dad cuts up dead bodies' – which usually prevented any further questions. But, on the whole, it was much easier to explain that their mother was a GP who was specializing in dermatology than that their father was a forensic pathologist.

In a few years, Chris and Anna would both be off to university. It was hard to imagine them as independent people leading independent lives. It was hard to imagine they wouldn't need me any more. I determined that, although my new job would certainly be demanding, I should try to spend as much time with them as possible before they left.

## 27

Once I had started up the department I was back in the mortuary, and this became a busy, productive period. Other staff arrived. Rob Chapman, a friend and excellent pathologist from Guy's joined me, and two secretaries, Rhiannon Layne and Kathy Paylor. And so did two clinical forensic doctors, Debbie Rogers and Margaret Stark. They examined the living victims of crime, and they also looked after the medical needs of the people who had been arrested and detained in police cells. These were the first academic clinical forensic posts in the UK, a great asset to our embryonic department. In addition, we had a trainee pathologist. Very quickly, we became nationally and internationally recognized, and that meant we were busy almost at once.

Being boss gave me the chance, to some extent, to choose my cases. One very difficult area I would have liked to palm off onto my colleagues was the very area I'd been immersed in with my last case at Guy's – babies. But I could see that wasn't fair. Because now everything was changing in the pathology of child death, and this reflected society's changing attitude to children. I realized that now I probably would have given a different cause of death for the baby of that drunken mother.

From the early 1990s, the number of SIDS deaths – or deaths diagnosed as SIDS – significantly declined, and that decline has continued (the most recent statistics tell us that SIDS now accounts for only 0.27 deaths per 1,000 live births).

The improvement was largely due to the worldwide campaign (called 'Back to Sleep' in the UK) which persuaded parents to stop putting their babies face down in bed, as this had been identified as a major risk factor in SIDS. Other factors we knew of included adults in the house smoking, adults sleeping on the sofa or in bed with the baby (which could result in 'overlaying' or rolling onto the child), alcohol- or substance-abusing parents, too much bedding and too high a room temperature. With all this knowledge, and an education programme for parents, the numbers fell.

Numbers also fell because perceptions of SIDS changed, and consequently the fundamentals of its diagnosis. It was now sometimes referred to as a 'diagnostic dustbin' and guidelines for pathologists were tightened up. The thinking was that, before diagnosing SIDS, we should examine very carefully first the history – both the child's medical history and the caregiver's story of events – then the scene itself and finally the pathology of the deceased child. There isn't really any positive pathology for SIDS. It's a question of confirming the absence of every other possible cause of death.

And why, really, were guidelines tightening up and people talking about SIDS as a 'diagnostic dustbin'? Simply because many pathologists did not follow the criteria laid down for its use and gave it for any death they couldn't explain – and often these deaths were under-investigated by both the police and the pathologist. SIDS had become such a catch-all that there were now unpalatable suspicions. Could it be that some so-called SIDS cases might be acts of adults rather than God?

Those uncomfortable suspicions were rooted in the pioneering child-protection work of Professor David Southall and his colleagues. In the light of evidence he produced, it was hard not to face facts. He was involved in studies which not only identified Munchausen syndrome by proxy – parents with this mental disorder deliberately make their children ill in order to receive attention and support – but also produced irrefutable evidence through covert video surveillance that some parents certainly do attempt to injure or even kill their children for reasons that are unclear.

In his most famous investigation, thirty-nine children who had recurrent episodes of apparently life-threatening events, usually outside hospital but sometimes on a hospital ward, were referred to a specialist ward where they were secretly filmed. In thirty-three cases, these 'events' turned out to be induced by a parent. The covert footage showed incidents not just of emotional abuse but also poisoning, strangulation and, especially, suffocation. In fact, there were no fewer than thirty attempts at suffocation in just this small group.

Thanks to the surveillance, professional intervention protected the children. But between them those children had forty-one siblings, of whom twelve had died suddenly and unexpectedly. Once the parents were exposed, four actually admitted to killing eight of these siblings. When these 'sibling' cases were reviewed it was found that, in eleven of the twelve cases, the cause of death given by the pathologist who had performed the post-mortem was SIDS. In the twelfth case, the cause given had been gastroenteritis, but further investigation now revealed the child had been poisoned. Fifteen more of the forty-one siblings were later discovered to have suffered abuse.

Naturally, there was widespread shock at these findings and considerable disbelief. I feel, as a result of David Southall's work, we started to move out of an age of innocence. A lot of people, however, preferred innocence. It was hard to accept that there were children who needed protection from the very adults who should be protecting them.

Suspicion gradually became an almost routine response to the unexplained death of a baby, and that must have felt very unfair to the innocent. So unfair that David Southall faced vitriolic and vocal opposition. The ethics of his covert video surveillance of parents came in for particular criticism. I fear that, without it, he never would have been believed, so incredible did his results seem at that time.

Parents (as well as many police officers and even social workers) who had once regarded any concern from outside the family for the welfare of children as an invasion of privacy, were now forced to accept change. Adult victims of all sorts of parental abuse were talking publicly about their childhoods and a light was shining onto family secrets in a way that had been impossible when privacy was king. That light was held by professionals working with children – health visitors, doctors, nursery staff – who were now encouraged to report any suspicions of abuse.

\*

As child protection became a subject for national debate, the discussion about unexplained baby deaths left theory behind and became concentrated in the specifics of just one case. I am talking about the trial of Sally Clark.

SIDS had once taken a cruel harvest from right across the social spectrum, but as the middle classes became informed about risk factors and minimized them, SIDS began to look like something more likely to affect the poor. Until, in 1996, Sally Clark, a well-off, middle-class solicitor and policeman's daughter whose background and bearing reflected that of so many respectable, professional, working mothers, lost first one baby to SIDS. And then, in 1997, another.

The first baby, a boy, was eleven weeks old. Sally Clark's husband, Stephen, also a lawyer, was out at the office party when his wife found the baby unconscious. She called an ambulance, but for some reason she was unable to open the door when it arrived. The baby the paramedics discovered had no pulse and had been cyanosed – meaning his lips and fingers were blue – for some time. But he was only officially declared dead after an hour when resuscitation attempts failed.

The pathologist who conducted the subsequent postmortem was worried by particular injuries: a split and bruise at the top of the baby's mouth, inside the lips, and the absence of any obvious cause of death. He had these injuries photographed and it is very unfortunate that the photographer's camera was not working properly and the resulting pictures were of such poor quality that they were to prove absolutely unhelpful in the furore that followed. That was extreme bad luck: I've only come across such decisive camera failure one other time in my entire career.

When the pathologist discussed his worries with the police and the coroner's officer, he had to agree that the split inside the baby's lip could have been caused by the resuscitation attempt. In the case of these particular injuries, such a cause would be rare – damage to that part of the mouth is indicative of abuse – but it is certainly possible that they occurred during the frantic hour of resuscitation.

The police and the coroner's officer chose to believe the cause was the attempted resuscitation and there was no further investigation. They were dealing with a well-off, professional family, not the kind of criminals or child abusers they normally encountered.

The baby had been X-rayed and no broken bones found. The pathologist had taken histology samples and these were pretty much normal. All except for the very small possibility – certainly not a probability – of some increase of inflammatory cells in a sample from the lungs.

He might have exonerated the parents by giving SIDS. Or, in view of the baby's injuries, he might have aired the possibility of an unnatural death by giving 'Unascertained'. Times were changing fast but the fact is, in 1996 he may also have been working for a conservative, one might even say Luddite, coroner: in those days any lawyer or medical practitioner with a few years under their belt could become a coroner. I do not know the coroner involved in this case but many of them, exclusively those who did not have a medical qualification, were still struggling with the concept of SIDS because it was a cause of death based on no definable evidence. And some coroners also disliked the word 'Unascertained', particularly when applied to babies. They wanted to say kind, comforting things to grief-stricken parents, not, 'We don't know why your baby's dead.' Limitations like this could leave a pathologist in limbo.

For whatever reason, the pathologist seized on the slides from the lung sample with their suggestion of inflammation and decided that the baby had died of natural causes: in fact, lower respiratory tract infection. The child's death was treated as natural.

But the following year the Clarks' second baby died too. He had been a few weeks premature but he was fine now, at two months old. Sally Clark breast-fed him and supplemented that with bottled milk. One evening, her husband went to prepare a bottle for the night feed, leaving the mother to watch TV while the baby lay in his bouncy chair. When she saw that her son was limp, she called her husband and rang an ambulance. The paramedics found the baby dead.

The same pathologist was involved and this time discovered injuries that suggested to him this baby may have been shaken, perhaps on several occasions over several days. He believed he had found haemorrhages in the eyes and spinal cord as well as some abnormalities of the ribs which suggested that there had been previous fracture or trauma.

Sally Clark and her husband were arrested on suspicion of the murder of their second child and, while they were being interviewed about his death, the pathologist quite rightly went back to his report on the death of the first child. In this he was complying with Home Office guidelines, which state that 'if previously held conclusions can no longer be substantiated then any change of opinion must be promptly and clearly stated irrespective of any possible embarrassment'.

The pathologist did change his opinion and was to suffer prolonged and considerable embarrassment.

Examining the microscope slides once again which had, possibly but not probably, shown a lung inflammation in the first child, he decided that the cause of death he had previously given was entirely wrong. He decided that there was no inflammation. He had discovered blood in the baby's alveoli, but had not even mentioned it before. He later said he had assumed this was simply consistent with changes after death. But he had since found that the nature of this finding might be abnormal and that it was consistent with asphyxiation.

At this point, as many experts subsequently pointed out, he might have kept the question open by revising the cause of death from 'Lower Respiratory Tract Infection' to 'Unascertained'.

One expert witness explained in the later court case why he personally would have done this:

Unascertained . . . means that the child's death may have been natural but without explanation – perhaps what the jury knows as a cot death. Or it might be that the child died unnaturally but I can't find out why, or it might be the child died of a natural disease that I am not clever enough to diagnose and recognize . . .

But the pathologist did not choose 'Unascertained'. Instead he submitted a further statement saying that he no longer believed the first child had died of natural causes. The volte face concluded that: 'There is evidence he died from an asphyxial mechanism such as smothering.'

Six weeks after her arrest for the murder of her second son, Sally Clark was also arrested for the murder of her first. At her trial, the jury famously heard evidence from the paediatrician Professor Sir Roy Meadow, who had popularized, if he did not actually coin, the maxim, 'One sudden infant death in a family is a tragedy, two is suspicious and three is murder unless proved otherwise.'

A memorable statistic was unfortunately added at Sally Clark's trial which was to become associated with Professor Meadow for ever: 'The chance of two children dying naturally in these circumstances is very, very long odds indeed. One in 73 million . . .'

One in 73 million was a headline grabber and may have sealed the defendant's fate. He went on to say, '. . . it's the chance of backing that long-odds outsider at the Grand National . . . let's say it's an 80 to 1 chance, you backed the winner last year, then the next year there's another horse at 80 to 1 and you back it again and it wins . . . you know, to get to these odds of 73 million you've got to back that 1 in 80 chance four years running.'

Sally Clark was found guilty by a jury majority of ten to two of both murders and sentenced to life imprisonment.

I was not directly involved in this case. But it affected all of us. Her conviction, and David Southall's work, was indicating that the murder of babies was much more common than we had all assumed and parents who murder their children are more common than we would have thought possible. Even 'nice', middle-class professional parents. We pathologists were called upon to offer a medical and scientific analysis within the context of society's current thinking and I'm sorry to tell you that the purity of scientific truth rarely cuts through contemporary social attitudes.

Personally, I could never forget how I had walked an endlessly wailing, lactose-intolerant baby around the house, night after night, thinking, in so far as one can think over the noise of penetrating screams, that I would do almost anything for some sleep. I knew that the middle classes, even without the pressures of poverty or isolation, were as vulnerable as other parents to extreme desperation.

Soon after Sally Clark's trial, a case of mine reflected what had now become the great controversy of child protection. When I saw this six-month-old baby in the mortuary he seemed to have been healthy and well cared for, but I was quickly aware of a distinctive triad of symptoms. He had a subdural haemorrhage, that is, a bleeding on the surface of the brain. The brain itself was swollen. And his eyes had haemorrhages in the retinas. These three symptoms, particularly without external signs of injury, were now regarded as the classic triad of symptoms of what was then called 'shaken baby syndrome'.

In the 1940s a radiologist, John Caffey, reported multiple fractures of varying ages in some children and initially thought this was a new disease. Later research showed the fractures were due to repeated trauma and in the 1960s the term 'battered baby syndrome' was first used. Then, in the 1970s, a neurological variant, shaken baby syndrome, was recognised as a form of whiplash by neurosurgeon Norman Guthkelch. So these syndromes, and their root cause in deliberately inflicted trauma, were medically well-known. However, they were only brought to public attention in 1997 by the famous case of the medical couple in Massachusetts who had left their baby in the care of a nineteen-year-old English au pair.

When the baby suddenly became ill and was rushed to hospital, he showed that classic triad of symptoms and, in a televised court case that obsessed America, young Louise Woodward was found guilty of murder. Many Americans were outraged when this charge was changed afterwards by the judge to manslaughter because he felt that there really was not sufficient evidence beyond reasonable doubt for a murder conviction. And that was because medical experts were so divided about shaken baby syndrome.

This was not the end of the story because by now shaken baby syndrome itself had become the story. Most people had never heard of it before Louise Woodward's trial and suddenly it was in the headlines and every pathologist was on full alert for the now-famous triad of symptoms.

In fact, as a cause of death it was then and is now highly controversial and the subject of much scientific and medical argument. Shaken baby syndrome, now also called abusive head injury or non-accidental head injury, has created its own angry groups of protesters and deniers. There is an ongoing search for natural causes to explain it.

Long after Sally Clark's imprisonment, in 2009, the Royal College of Pathologists attempted to bring together the various sides of the debate and this disparate group was able to issue a statement on what they called traumatic head injury (which was yet another name for just the same thing) reminding pathologists that, even if all elements of the triad are present, each may have other, non-traumatic causes. The statement said clearly that the triad alone is not enough to say a parent harmed a baby 'beyond reasonable doubt': more evidence would be needed for that. And special care should be taken interpreting the injuries when the baby is under three months old, because they might, possibly, have been caused during birth.

It looked like a consensus. However, if anything, the debate became more heated. Forty years after first describing the features of this particular type of head injury, Norman Guthkelch in 2012 reviewed its history and expressed concern:

> While society is rightly shocked by an assault on its weakest members and demands retribution, there seem to have been instances in which medical science and the law has gone too far in hypothesizing and criminalizing alleged acts of violence in which the only evidence has been the presence of the classic triad or even just one or two of its elements.

At the end of the 1990s, shaken baby syndrome was very firmly on the pathologist's radar and the six-month-old baby I saw seemed to show every relevant symptom. According to his mother, however, he had launched himself from his car seat, which she had placed on a work surface, with no prior warning that he was physically capable of doing such a thing. As a result, he had fallen out of the seat and about one metre down onto a hard kitchen floor. Even a few years earlier, I would have been reluctant to believe her. But, post-Woodward, I had very grave concerns indeed.

The mother came from an impoverished and war-torn nation and had been brought by her husband to live in London with his mother and various other family members. She spoke no English. Their accommodation was overcrowded. She still had a relationship with her husband but, because there was so little room in the family flat, had recently begun to live separately in housing that had, it seemed, been provided by the council. Her flat was clean and airy but apart from a bed and a television, she had no furniture and evidently just sat on the floor.

She seemed to spend all day there alone. Outside the family, whom she seldom saw, she only knew one person in London and that friend lived far away. I thought of my desperation with the wailing baby Chris all those years ago and pitied this woman for the utter isolation in which she lived, far from home, with this small baby.

She had no car, of course, but carried her son around the flat in his car seat. When she made meals, she took him to the kitchen and perched his seat on the work surface. He was not strapped in. One evening she was busy preparing the food, heard a loud thump ('a sickening thud', are words which often seem to crop up in court), and turned around to find the baby face-down on the floor. He cried immediately but his eyes rapidly became staring and his breathing erratic: it was clear something was very wrong.

She tried to phone 999 but was unable to make herself understood. She tried to phone her husband, who spoke English, but the emergency services were still blocking the line. She ran down to the street to get someone else to phone 999 but by that time the police had already responded to her distressed although incomprehensible call.

They found a baby with blood coming from his nose and mouth, shaking slowly and losing consciousness. The police would not let the mother get into the ambulance and the baby was rushed to hospital in an apparently deteriorating condition. CT scans revealed severe internal injuries, but initially it seemed he would probably survive. However, his cardiovascular system became unstable and, in spite of all attempts at resuscitation, he died twelve hours after his mother had called the emergency services.

So far as we know, natural causes for the three individual symptoms which are together suggestive of shaken baby syndrome (like blood clotting difficulties) are very rare. While one should always be alert for these rare natural causes, I felt that a bleeding, swollen brain and bleeding retinas indicated that the baby had received a major trauma. Sometimes that trauma may be an accident, like a car crash. And sometimes, particularly if there are no external marks, it is not an accident.

In this case, I was further convinced that the baby had been shaken because, despite the internal haemorrhages, there was no fracture of the skull, no bruising of the head, no trauma at all on the outside to show that he had plummeted from a work surface onto a hard floor. He had the triad, although no trauma to the spinal cord at the neck, which is another associated symptom.

The mother was tried for manslaughter. The defence pathologist felt that the baby's injuries meant he had been subjected to either an acceleration-deceleration trauma (shaking) or a head impact. He did agree that, in a six-month-old baby, shaking is the most common cause of such internal injuries, and added that it is sometimes unclear whether shaking or impact is the more important factor, since babies who are shaken are then sometimes thrown forcefully down. However, his overall opinion was that the brain swelling alone had killed this baby, and that the injuries therefore confirmed the mother's story.

Appearing for the prosecution, I had briefed counsel on this and pointed out the lack of bruising or external mark at all resulting from the alleged fall. When this was put to the defence pathologist he cited the famous case of a two-year-old who fell off a stool just about half a metre high in McDonald's and died because her brain was so swollen – with no obvious external injuries.

The jury decided that the mother in this case was not guilty of manslaughter. She walked free.

A year later she had another son. The local authority knew that she had been acquitted, but they believed there was still enough evidence to suggest that the next child might not be safe in her hands. They set in motion care proceedings to remove the new baby.

In the Crown Court, a mother charged with man-slaughter would be convicted only if her guilt is *beyond reasonable doubt*. The Family Court, which hears the local authority's request to remove her next child from her, must reconsider her case all over again – but apply a different level of proof. The Family Court applies the lower standard of proof – *the balance of probabilities* – to reach its conclusions. That can be defined as a 50.1 per cent chance of guilt – a 'lower' standard of proof than the standard of proof that is beyond reasonable doubt. So, different courts can reach different conclusions based on the different levels of proof they require, and it often happens that the Crown Court does not have enough evidence to convict for the death of a child but the Family Court feels there is sufficient evidence to remove the living sibling of that child. And so, truth, that elastic commodity I once thought so immutable, becomes a question not of fact but of definition.

No one can be criminally convicted because they are guilty 'on the balance of probabilities'. Even if the Family Court decides, using this definition of guilt, that a parent has 'most probably' killed their child, the parent is free. And, because these courts are entirely closed to press and public, no one will ever know. Although they might be aware that the court has ordered any surviving or future children be taken away, or that some other safeguarding option has been chosen for them. The Family Court's sole aim is not to jail parents, it is to safeguard children, and that is what happened in the case of the woman who said her child had fallen from his car seat.

For pathologists, the chasm between two courts and two standards of guilt can be a nightmare. According to our evidence about the death of a first child, innocent, bereaved parents may never be allowed to keep future children. Or alternatively, we may be exposing a second child to a killer parent.

The universal tendency to leniency where mothers are concerned, of which everyone, including me early in my career, has been guilty, is a symptom of the deep human compassion most people feel for parents under pressure. I only have to think of baby Chris to feel that same compassion right now. If poverty had been knocking at my door, debts climbing in the window, chaos pervading every air molecule in the house, would I have been able to bridle my exasperation? Without the luxury of a quiet place to escape to in the house, would I have been able to stop exhaustion and strain spilling into fury?

Compassion certainly has its place but, in the case of child abuse, we must extend our compassion to those who may not yet even be born. When society, when pathologists, finally realized how widespread child murder and abuse was, each baby death assumed a double importance. Justice for the deceased, yes. But the safety of other children in the family became paramount. Our tendency to leniency no longer had a place.

Sometimes, a year or more after a baby has been buried, we return to the file because another child has been born and there is the question now of safeguarding the living. By that time, a fuller picture of the baby's life and death may have emerged. Parents' abusive, neglectful or simply absent care may have been exposed or histories uncovered. The whole case has a new slant. So we reopen the file and review it. Of all the files I revisit, baby cases, that minefield of moral and emotional ordnance, are the ones I examine and re-examine the most. When I moved to St George's I would have liked simply to avoid them, but as the 1990s wore on it became obvious that the question of babies and why they died was at the heart of forensic pathology and must be addressed by everyone, including me.

# 28

There was another change in our profession, one that seemed to accelerate at an alarming rate when I arrived at St George's: the stress involved in court appearances.

Forensic pathologists of the past were household names and every newspaper reader between the wars knew who Sir Bernard Spilsbury was: a sort of Sherlock Holmes figure whose brilliant analysis of any case ensured that, if he were appearing for the prosecution, the defendant would be hanged. Long after his death, the icon's cases were re-examined and his logic found sometimes to be less than Holmesian. But at the time it was unthinkable to challenge him.

His successor was my own hero, Professor Keith Simpson. Simpson – whom, at the end of his career and beginning of mine, I had actually breathlessly watched carrying out a post-mortem – was a man with far more humanity and humour than Spilsbury. But he, too, operated in the days when the expert witness was held in such regard that he was rarely challenged.

In my early years of practice, court appearances hadn't been too bad. In the first months I avoided controversial cases if I could, although it was hard to know in advance what would turn into a circus. In general, counsel just wanted the facts from the pathologist: there was then still, if not the respect of earlier ages, at least its residue.

However, by the time I reached St George's, barristers had begun to see post-mortem reports as a possible chink in the opposition's armour and more and more regarded the testimony of the expert witness as an opportunity to stick the knife into the other side. Some pathologists enjoy this. For anyone with macho pretensions, courtroom barracking is the professional equivalent of a Saturday night fight and there are many who are ready to roll up their sleeves. Watching their courtroom appearances would leave me open-mouthed and incredulous.

QC: Do you mean to tell me that you are absolutely sure that the knife wounds were inflicted while the deceased was lying down?

CONFIDENT COLLEAGUE: I do.

QC: You are certain?

CC: I am.

QC: But are you aware that we have heard from two witnesses that he was last seen walking down the Old Kent Road?

CC: I am aware of all witness statements.

QC: Then will you perhaps entertain the possibility he –?

CC: I will not.

QC: You will not even say there is a possibility that –?

CC: I am sorry that I have to remind you I have sworn an oath today. An oath to tell the whole truth and nothing but the truth. Therefore, you can produce a witness saying the deceased was playing premier league football or that he was walking down the Old Kent Road or anything at all, but it is still my

duty, my oath, my role as an expert witness, to tell
the truth and only the truth as I see it. (*sonorously*)
And therefore I tell you that this man was stabbed
as he lay on his back.

How I envied that colleague. I knew I could never
be like him. In those circumstances I cannot but admit
the possibility, however slim, that I may be wrong, that
there are other explanations, other versions of the truth.
While my job requires me, at the same time, to insist that
I have reached the correct conclusion.

My favourite court was the one that, in theory at least,
is non-adversarial and informal: the coroner's court. Here,
the coroner is leading an inquiry into the truth. Here is
the deceased's wife, sitting an arm's length away, red-eyed,
anxious for the truth but fearing it, still shocked many
months after the death. Here are the deceased's children,
tearful, angry, telling the coroner they don't think it was
an accident and they have a good idea who was involved.
Here are his friends, awkward, supportive, overawed by
the court setting.

I turn to the relatives in order to explain, as simply,
kindly, clearly as I can, causing as little pain as possible,
how the deceased's life ended. I answer their questions. I
nod sympathetically. Often, they ask the same questions
again and again as if they can't hear the answers, no matter how hard they listen. The coroner thanks me and I
return to my seat.

As I leave, some relatives catch me to ask the same
questions. Again. I tell them once more that he really
didn't suffer, the end came quickly, he probably did not

have time to comprehend what was happening, he was otherwise in good health, no, there was no evidence of cancer and the chest pains he used to complain of were not caused by heart disease.

Usually, the coroner then reaches a verdict. Accidental death, suicide, natural causes, misadventure, unlawful killing . . . the relatives leave feeling emotionally exhausted but with a sense that death's formalities are all over now. They have listened and have, hopefully, been listened to. The deceased's case has been fully examined in public and the reason for and fact of his passing officially stated.

If only the criminal courts had the same degree of humanity. There are few jobs where it is routine to stand up in public and defend your professional opinion in the face of very personal attack. There are, of course, expert witnesses who get the reputation of being a liar for hire. I'm not one of them and don't like to be treated that way by solicitors asking if I might alter my view a little or delete an inconvenient paragraph in my report. When I chose this career, I thought that I would be conveying the truth about the dead to the living – who would be grateful to hear it. But, as we approached the new century, I instead was starting to feel like the faithful dog that proudly lays a stick at the feet of his master only to receive a hearty kick for his efforts.

Despite all this, I usually go to court feeling confident. I know my subject, I know my findings, I know my conclusions. But, once in the witness box under oath, I have no control over events. The barristers are in control, and when they say I must stay and answer questions, if there is no intervention from the judge, then stay I must.

Not long into my time at St George's, I had an experience in the witness box which was so unpleasant that it gave me many sleepless nights and seemed to point at things to come. I had no idea, when I performed the post-mortem on a 'rent boy', or teenage male prostitute, that this case would not be straightforward. He had been found the night before and had died in hospital. His body looked extraordinary. He was covered in livid bruises, and I do mean covered. He was virtually a definition of that old threat adults shouted at naughty children in my day, 'I'll beat you black and blue!'

I counted 105 bruises and many, many abrasions. The weapon used was a cylindrical metal bar from a set of weights. The bar had cross-hatching at the ends, which was reproduced in some of the wounds. There were abrasions also, where, it seemed to me, the circular end of the metal bar had been used in a sort of stabbing action.

It is unusual for someone to die of bruising, but the nineteen-year-old victim had sustained a remarkable number of blows. I gave the cause of death as multiple blunt trauma. In fact, once the patient arrived in A&E he developed a disorder called disseminated intravascular coagulation, which arises from the overactivation of the body's defence system against trauma: this results in the blood-clotting mechanisms being overwhelmed and so further, almost continuous, bleeding takes place everywhere, including from vital organs. Shock follows and, in many cases, death.

I went to the block of flats where the events took place. The young man had been found on the third floor, but he had been beaten on the ninth floor, so he had somehow staggered down seventy-four stairs before collapsing. I measured the steps and the risers but it was clear to me that his injuries, except possibly for one or two where he had stumbled on the stairs, were caused because he had been beaten by the iron bar, and not because he had fallen downstairs.

The defendant, also a male prostitute, also about nineteen years old, was actually the deceased's best friend, and they shared the same 'uncle' who pimped them or funded them or both. It has amazed me, over the years, how frequently men (but not noticeably women) will kill their best friend. And brothers commit fratricide even more frequently. In this case, the deceased went to the defendant's flat. They drank all afternoon and evening: the dead lad's extrapolated blood alcohol levels were around twice the drink-drive limit. It was just before midnight that a resident on the third floor called an ambulance: she had found the victim lying injured outside her flat. He was taken to hospital but died less than twelve hours later.

What had happened?

In my opinion the friend started to hit the deceased and just could not stop. Eventually, the deceased escaped from his flat and down the stairs. If his attacker had reasoned at all he had probably reasoned that no one ever dies of thumps and bruises – which is a fallacy.

I received notification that I was being called by the prosecution as an expert witness. That was routine. And it felt like a routine case. I did learn that the defence barrister was one I recognized, a particularly persistent tiger. An old tiger, actually. But not without teeth. He was known for stalking expert witnesses but I was still not really concerned. The case was quite straightforward and I'd probably be in and out of the witness box in a few hours.

At a pre-trial conference with the prosecution, counsel had warned me that he would be going through each of the 105 injuries with me. I hoped that after such a marathon it would be so obvious to the jury why the young man had died that the defence would have no further questions and I would be allowed to go.

I took the stand and made my oath. The court had been supplied with copies of some of the post-mortem photos: not as sanitized as the cartoonish images we use today, but nothing too horrific, and each area of bruising was documented and numbered. I had prepared these photographic exhibits and given them to the Crown Prosecution Service well in advance, but, as usual where pictures are concerned, there was a lot of bumbling about. Officials stumbled blindly here and there with the wrong pictures, judge and jury found they had different ones, people passed pictures to other people and I had to suppress hysterical laughter at the sheer disorganization of it all.

Prosecuting counsel began by lulling everyone to sleep as we discussed in detail, as previously agreed, each one of the 105 injuries. In the course of this, I made two small errors, both picked up in a kindly way by prosecuting counsel. The first was on injury 11 on the right-hand side of the back.

ME: . . . indicating that once again that injury has been caused by a linear blunt object of similar size to the object that caused the injuries on the left-hand side of the chest.

QC: When you refer to the chest, you mean the back?

ME: Oh, I do apologize, yes I did. Those injuries I have just been talking about are the highlighted injuries to the back.

A daft error. And idiotic when I did it again, much later:

ME: ... and as you can see, injury 71 is a ten by three centimetres deep bruise.

QC: Now, did you not, in your report, in addition to those numbered injuries, find something else here?

ME: Indeed, once again as with the chest, I found some area of parallel bruising over the legs.

QC: As with the back?

ME: As with the back. I am sorry. You are quite right, I am confusing the back and the chest. Over the back were, at least, three areas of parallel bruising...

Considering the enormity of the crime we were discussing, these mistakes seemed small enough. I said back when I meant chest and was corrected. I don't think I confused the judge, jury, prosecution or defendant. Counsel for the defence, however, must have been rubbing his hands.

When the judge asked the defence how long their questions would take, because he was deciding when to give the jury a break, the old tiger said, rather ominously, that, since new material had just emerged, it would perhaps be better to have the break now.

There was a twenty-minute pause, one that chess players might regard as strategic. I spent it wondering just what the new information was. Was it something I had said? I remembered defence counsel's reputation and, sure enough, within a few minutes of our return . . .

> Defence QC: You have, I think, on two occasions, referred to the chest when you meant the back?

Oh-oh. When a QC tries to catch me out on small and insignificant errors to prove to the jury my incompetence early in the cross-examination, then I know that there's trouble ahead.

> ME: I did indeed, yes.
>
> QC: That is a mistake that can be easily made, can it not?
>
> ME: Well, yes, it is easy to confuse these things. I tend to consider the back of the chest and the front of the chest.
>
> QC: But, Dr Shepherd, that is not what you said.
>
> ME: No. I mistakenly said chest when I meant back.
>
> QC: Quite a mistake in its way, is it not?
>
> ME: Well, it is a mistake. I'm not sure how 'quite' a mistake it is.
>
> QC: Very well. When you are more precise though, perhaps you expect a higher degree of accuracy. For example, the weight of the metal bar (*referring to the murder weapon here*) – 450 grams. Is that right?
>
> ME: That is what my notes say.

QC: Well, we shall be hearing, no doubt, an admission of evidence that it was 421 grams. Not a great deal turns on the weight, except the accuracy of what you say.

I felt myself turning red at this point. Confusing chest and back wasn't serious but being accused of getting the weight of the alleged murder weapon wrong might look careless to a jury. No time to think about it; defence counsel, without warning, entirely changed subject.

QC: If a man had some drink – it all depends how much, and whether he is accustomed to it – it may affect his steadiness of gait?

ME: It may.

QC: And, if he has suffered some physical trauma – blows – that will not improve matters, will it?

ME: Well, I think that depends on the blows he has received.

QC: Now, Dr Shepherd, you said the deceased had received about a hundred blows, is that right?

ME: *(very carefully now)* That is . . . an approximation.

QC: Now follow this through as a logical thought, would you please. You are a doctor, called to a flat on the ninth floor. You have been told and you can see a man has had . . . let us take your evidence at full strength . . . 105 blows. He says, 'I want to walk down to the third floor. I know I had a drink.' There are seventy-four steps and eight and a half landings. Would you say, 'All right, old boy, get going. I'll see you at the bottom?'

If I hadn't been under oath and giving evidence, I might have laughed. Would the QC, on finding himself on the ninth floor of a block of flats with a drunken young male prostitute, really address him as 'old boy'? But the real concern for me was: where was this going?

After an endless series of further questions about if, how and why I would help a drunken rent boy down the stairs in the middle of the night, the QC exploded in a manner oddly reminiscent of my father.

QC: Can I come straight to the heart of the matter and not pussyfoot around answering and questioning? You would have wanted to make sure he did not fall down the stairs – seventy-four of them – would you not?

ME: That would be one of my concerns, yes.

QC: Yes. Because if a man had been subjected to the number of blows you indicated, he might fall?

ME: Clearly, anyone in that circumstance might fall.

QC: Thank you. If he fell on uncarpeted stairs, he might injure himself?

ME: Certainly, a fall onto the lower stairwell I saw could result in injury, yes.

QC: Yes!

Good heavens. Surely the defence was not going to argue that the 105 injuries were virtually all caused by the victim falling downstairs? Surely he would not try to persuade the jury that this was not a murder with the metal bar but just an unlucky series of falls? The idea was absurd.

Counsel asked me to describe the stairwell in minute detail, although in fact the jury had been given pictures of it. I lost count of the number of times he repeated how many stairs there were. I think everyone in court must have dreamed about the number 74 that night. And a fall down these seventy-four concrete stairs, he kept insisting, could be very serious. I was unable to contradict him. But I didn't believe the deceased's injuries, or at least the fatal ones, resulted from falling downstairs.

Then he went back to the injuries. Individually. Again. All 105 of them. One by one, he asked me to prove they had not been caused by the deceased's alleged fall, and one by one he challenged each answer.

This cross-examination amazed me. The deceased had been a drifter who had lived most of his childhood in and out of care, had probably spent at least some of his subsequent time living on the streets and had recently been released from jail. The defendant's background was very similar. If either one had ever received a fraction of the public money, care and interest that was devoted to this trial then I doubt there would have been a murder.

As for the defence barrister, it was good he was working so hard to defend a client who was clearly from the margins of society. Had he ever passed the lad huddled in a doorway, I don't expect learned counsel would have looked at him, let alone thrown a coin in his cup. But now the young man was on trial for murder, legal arguments about him consumed the barrister. I wished he could do his job without attacking my reputation as an expert witness. But I knew that in another case and with another jury we might be on the same side and then, instead of excoriating me, he would be praising my experience and skills.

The cross-examination continued for the rest of the day and then carried on the next morning. And the next afternoon. And the following morning. Now the defence QC wasn't just arguing that the injuries were caused by falling downstairs but that the cross-hatching from the surface of the iron bar reproduced on the victim's skin was actually simply caused by the warp and weft of his cotton T-shirt.

Then, many tea breaks later, as I returned to the witness box ready for a few more rounds with my back against the ropes, I watched him bounce in, a spring in his step and his eyes darting dangerously beneath his wig. I knew the tiger was planning to pounce.

QC: Alcohol, I suppose, if you are affected by it, will make you, perhaps, slightly more liable to bleed than would otherwise be the case?

ME: In the chronic alcoholic whose damaged liver may have blood-clotting problems, yes. But I found nothing to suggest that is the case here. I believe alcohol would have a very minimal effect.

QC: Do you know anything about that as a clinician?

ME: No, I do not.

QC: Not aware of that?

ME: Not particularly.

QC: What do you mean, not particularly? Are you aware of it?

ME: I am not aware, throughout my experience, of anyone who has suffered significantly more bruising when they are under the influence of alcohol than someone who is sober.

That was not the answer counsel wanted to hear. He argued and argued with me that alcohol dilated the tiny blood vessels on the surface of the skin – which I agreed with – and therefore that drinkers were much more vulnerable to bruising – which I did not. I lost count of the number of times he took me, step by step, through his logical but erroneous deduction that the victim was covered in bruises simply because he had been drinking. I really began to doubt who had been beaten by an iron bar, the victim or me, but I stuck steadfastly to scientific fact. Finally, the QC exploded.

QC: Where do you get this from? Can you do some research overnight?

ME: I can consult the preclinical medical textbooks about the effects of trauma on the skin.

QC: What book do you suggest I consult overnight?

ME: I would suggest you consult any molecular biology book, I'm afraid I cannot give you a name.

QC: Aren't you familiar with any?

ME: Perhaps a textbook by Guyton will help, I cannot tell you which edition is current, I think the third or fourth edition. Or any haematology textbook will cover it.

QC: Any haematology author you can name?

ME: Not specifically, no.

JUDGE: How many pages is counsel likely to have to read, Dr Shepherd?

ME: I'm afraid I cannot help you with that.

QC: It is beyond me, but I shall still have a look.

JUDGE: Yes, and pass it to me afterwards, please, Counsel.

QC: I will, M'Lud.

By now I hated both the QC and the judge and suspected that they were members of the same chambers, or at least the same London club. Once, when the judge showed impatience with the defence, the QC asked to speak to him without the jury present. The jury, press, public and I filed dutifully out of the courtroom. When counsel and judge are talking in this way it usually means that a point of law is being argued and, on returning, there is a distinctly chilly atmosphere in the court, with one barrister smiling and the other sulking. But these QCs and this judge were all smiling happily when we returned, like pals at a fireside.

The defence was trying to explain away the horrific beating the dead lad had received by persuading the jury he had fallen downstairs (did I mention that there were seventy-four stairs?) and in the course of this he had become so badly bruised because he'd had a few drinks. I spent the evening feverishly phoning friends to discuss bruising and searching the hospital library for that textbook.

The next day we were at it again. It was all I could do to contain my own homicidal feelings.

Defence QC: You referred me and the court to a textbook. Guyton.

ME: Indeed.

QC: Have you got it with you now?

ME: I have a copy now.

QC: Do you have the passage you relied upon?

ME: I have marked the page that deals with what happens in the body following damage to a blood vessel.

QC: You've got it there?

ME: Yes, in this particular edition it is chapter 36.

QC: Which edition?

ME: I believe the eighth.

QC: Hmm. You had, of course, referred us to the third or fourth edition.

ME: I think I said I did not know which edition is most current.

QC: May I see it?

But I think he had already seen a copy. He asked me endless questions about platelets and clotting in an attempt to prove his point until the jury was nodding off and even the judge interrupted.

JUDGE: Please forgive me, but what I would like to ask Dr Shepherd is: this chapter you referred to – is there something in there which actually says alcohol increases bruising?

ME: It is the absence in that book, M'Lud, and in other books I have consulted, of anything saying alcohol causes increased bruising. It is the absence of those facts.

JUDGE: Because, if this was a sustainable proposition, you would expect to find it in that book, at that chapter?

ME: I would indeed, M'Lud.

That didn't really stop the defence. The QC made his false point in a variety of ways, once, twice, three times more, that alcohol increases capillary blood flow and so bruising must be more likely.

A whole week after I took the witness stand, I was allowed to go. What a relief.

This case illustrates that there are facts – and there are the conclusions that can be drawn from them. In the adversarial cauldron of that courtroom, truth had turned into an individual, nuanced, malleable commodity, and that is why as an expert witness I was pressured to interpret facts in ways I found uncomfortable. Advocacy – the art of a lawyer making his case – need have no conscience and any Bar school would agree that some good cases are lost by poor advocacy and that some poor cases are won by good advocacy. Overall, the balance of justice relies on a concept that has served our society well for centuries: that twelve people drawn randomly and with no special training can listen to and form a judgement based on all the evidence they hear.

In this case, the jury found the defendant guilty of murder and he went to jail. I wonder if he had as many sleepless nights as I did. But at least it was over.

Except it wasn't. After his client had spent a couple of years in jail, the barrister sought leave to appeal against the conviction because he had new evidence. The new evidence was that I had failed to produce any textbook in court which would contradict the QC's theory that alcohol intake was responsible for the deceased's bruising after he fell downstairs. And he listed a number of other ways in which I had allegedly been incompetent.

Now I certainly began to wonder who was being tried: me or the convicted murderer. But I did have time to muster some support. A very senior haematologist read the trial transcript and wrote a report, which concluded: 'Alcohol-induced skin capillary flow would have played at most a trivial role in the skin haemorrhage (bruising). This spectacular red herring was pressed hard by the defence in the name of common sense but the image conjured up, of vessels bloated with blood, is misleading.'

We spent quite a lot of time hanging around the Court of Appeal before the defence's case was heard. Then it was all over in an instant. The spurious 'new evidence' had been seen by their lordships for what it was and leave to appeal was not granted.

I admire the persistence of that QC in fighting for his client, a very disadvantaged young man. If I were ever accused of murder, then I would want him defending me. As an expert witness in his firing line, however, I felt he had shown a remarkable ability to ride roughshod over medical facts which did not favour his case.

Since then, if I am in court and the going gets tough, my coping mechanism is Alexander Pope. The lines my father wrote so painstakingly for me in that dictionary all those years ago instructed me to speak diffidently even when sure I am right, to readily admit the possibility that I may be wrong, to examine my errors and admit to them, to teach or correct others with generous regard for their feelings, never to agree for politeness' sake with concepts I know are wrong and to accept correction when it is appropriate. Despite the aggression and single-mindedness our adversarial system fosters, and its frequent disregard for the truth, I try to hold to Pope's principles.

## 29

Just thinking about the Hyde area of Manchester always gives me a warm glow. It was here that my mother had been brought up, it was here that her family and friends had lived. It was a place of happy visits when I was small and a place of pilgrimage all my life, too, because my mother was buried here.

It pleased me to think of the old ladies who came from Hyde – my grandmother, my aunt – who were so unlike the isolated, undernourished elderly people whose bodies I sometimes saw. They always welcomed me with warm and caring arms, drawing me into their busy lives and polished homes. They were noticeably an intrinsic part of a wider community.

In 1998 I received a call from a defence solicitor asking me to perform a second post-mortem examination on just such a lady from just that area. Mrs Kathleen Grundy had been known to my mother's family as a friend and schoolmate of my aunt. She had died on 24 June and on 1 July she had been buried in the same cemetery as my mother.

In August, however, she had been exhumed and now I stood over her body in the mortuary of Tameside General Hospital.

She was eighty-one but appeared to have been in exceptionally good health. There were no signs of a struggle.

And, unusually for anyone her age and for the next generation too, her arteries showed only minimal atheroma.

But toxicology told a different story. Although I could find no injection site on her body, she had evidently consumed a substantial dose of morphine or diamorphine in the hours leading up to her death. I gave as its cause: overdose of morphine.

In fact, she had died at the hands of her trusted family doctor, and it was through her sudden death that Harold Shipman was finally revealed as a serial killer. He was highly regarded by his patients, discussed and admired in that community I remembered with such fondness. Many described him as the nicest doctor in the area. He was especially loved by the elderly because he was happy to make home visits and, having worked in Hyde for some time, when he set up his own practice in 1992 he was inundated with patients by word-of-mouth recommendation.

Suspicions about him were aroused by Kathleen Grundy's sudden death just days after her will had apparently been changed to favour him. He had certified her cause of death as: 'Old Age'.

Further cases were immediately opened and more exhumations followed. I attended five of these postmortems. The next I saw, a seventy-three-year-old, had very mild coronary disease and mild emphysema. She cannot have had pneumonia, as claimed by Shipman on her death certificate. She did, however, have morphine poisoning. The next body told the same story. They all did.

It seemed frankly incredible that a family doctor could have killed six of his patients. In a letter I wrote afterwards I said:

It is clearly essential that the source of the morphine is identified and the possibility of contamination must also be considered ... given the delay between death and post-mortem examinations and the numerous events and actions that have surrounded these bodies, the possibility of contamination needs to be positively excluded ... I would suggest that advice is sought from a chemist to see if it is possible for chemicals used in the manufacture of embalming fluid, coffin wood or coffin furniture to be contaminated by substances containing morphine whilst buried ... finally, the possibility of other links between the bodies should also be explored (embalmers, undertakers, staff).

Of course, I thought every other possibility should be investigated not just because I was pathologist for Shipman's defence (yes, even serial killers are entitled to a defence) but because I was, we all were, resistant to the idea that a doctor had systematically killed his patients. A few years later, when Shipman had been imprisoned for the murder of no fewer than fifteen patients, it was hard to stomach the conclusions of Dame Janet Smith's public inquiry – that he had, over more than twenty years, certainly killed 215 people and there were hundreds more cases for which it was impossible at this stage to ascertain the facts.

His reasons are unclear. Generally, his victims lived alone. Generally, but not always, they were elderly. Generally, but not always, they were women. Anybody hoping that Shipman would eventually reveal the reasons for his actions – and perhaps confirm how many of the 494 deaths which had occurred on his watch he had actually caused – had their hopes dashed a few years later, in 2004, when he was found hanging in his cell.

Hyde changed for me after the exhumations. Instead of being a place I associated with my mother's family warmth and bustling old ladies, it became a place where old ladies lay dead at the hands of a serial killer they had trusted to take care of them.

When I returned to London from the exhumations, still half disbelieving that small part of Shipman's crimes we then suspected, I had another unpleasant experience: I crossed swords with Iain West. To my amazement, he had retired from Guy's. After all those years of swearing he would never stop, he had done just that. The rumour was that Iain was unwell but, of course, it was impossible for him to disappear from the London murder scene and just tend his garden in Sussex. He popped up frequently in the mortuary and in court, and when I returned from Manchester, brooding over the unfolding truth about Shipman, I found that he was to be my adversary in a knifing case.

We disagreed fundamentally: not by meeting face to face but by writing strongly worded, contradictory reports. His rebuttal was, as usual, extremely robust. Although it did occur to me at the time, and not just in retrospect, that his prose was a little less robust than it used to be.

The case centred on the perpetrator's account of how the knife entered the heart of the victim. Such accounts are often highly creative and by now I think I had heard every excuse in the book for the presence of a blade in another person's body. The most common is the claim that 'he ran onto the knife'. This is not always easy to prove or disprove and I need as many witness accounts as possible to help me reconstruct the attack. On this occasion, there were none. A woman and her husband had argued, the outcome was his death, and we only had her word to go on. The senior investigating officer actually phoned me for advice before interviewing her, a rare enough event, but he knew the entire case did rest on her exact description of what happened.

I said, 'Don't give me generalities, pin her down. Don't let her tell you: "He just came at me!" That means nothing, so get her to re-enact it, describe it, say who was where and how she was holding the knife, which hand did she have the knife in and in which direction each of them moved. Then I might be able to prove or disprove her story.'

He did exactly what I asked. This case, however, remained a conundrum.

The divorcing couple were arguing very acrimoniously over which of them their two young sons should live with. They were well off and their house was large and well cared for. The father wanted the two boys desperately and a Family Court hearing was imminent. They were all still living in the same house, although the mother had arranged to take a rental property for herself and the children which they would move into shortly.

On the day of his death, the father had taken time off work to go out with the children. The mother was waving them goodbye when he suddenly stopped the car in the driveway and went into the house, gesturing for the mother to follow him. Thinking he had forgotten something, she did so. The father shut the door behind them and announced that he wanted the children to live with him.

According to the wife's statement, here is the argument which followed:

I said: 'But you go to work, how are you going to do this?'

And he said: 'I'm going to resign. And I'm going to take care of my children.'

I said: 'Oh no you're not.'

The wife then described her husband's fury. Its tell-tale sign was the way he twisted his jaw: she remembered this from one previous occasion when he had hit her. But, as she made clear, despite the middle-class lifestyle she was a tough cookie from a tough area and had learned early in life that cowering only encourages bullies. So on that previous occasion she had hit him back and now she was ready to do the same.

She was unable to explain how the couple had moved from the hallway to the kitchen.

But the next thing was when I was at the back of the kitchen and I thought he was punching me in the stomach. He started punching me in the stomach and I thought he was hitting me but when I looked, I looked down and I saw a green handle and he wasn't punching me, it was stabbing me.

I said: 'What are you doing, you're trying to kill me!'

And he, then he got it, got the knife from my stomach and he started shoving it into my neck. He was trying to cut my throat. He was trying to get my artery cut in my throat so I would die . . .

And I said to him: 'For God's sake, you're trying to kill me, think about the boys . . . don't, don't kill me, think about the boys . . . you can have the boys . . . have the boys, just please don't kill me.'

It didn't occur to me that he might get another knife or anything but then he started kicking me. He got my head and banged my head on the floor. I got a bruise here and he broke a tooth. He's banging me and banging me and he got a kitchen chair and he hit me with the chair and I just thought, my God, he's not going to stop until I'm dead. I'm half dead already with all these wounds. I was soaked in blood. I felt like I'd, I'd, been in the shower I was so covered in blood.

He wasn't saying anything, he was just shoving it into my neck and I had to get that knife off of him . . . he was holding me here and shoving it into my neck and I, with my right hand, I got hold of the handle or the blade or whatever it was and I just held on to it . . . there was blood everywhere, all over the floor and the wall.

And I had, had, already had the knife in my hand, my right hand, so I swiped. I either went forward or I swiped with the knife . . . I must have either slipped or I went down on the floor and I was cowering over the knife . . .

The interviewer stopped her there and asked her to act out exactly what happened, more than once. He was able to establish that she had waved the knife in the air as she sat on the ground, but she was unable to describe the contact between the victim and the knife. Indeed, she had no reason to believe she had killed her husband because he ran out of the room. She rushed to the garage, locked the door and called the police. And throughout this, the two little boys were strapped into their car seats in front of the house.

Was she telling the truth? Or had she killed him and then injured herself to substantiate her story that he had attacked her?

Pictures of the scene confirmed her claim that there was blood on the kitchen walls and that it was thick on the floor. Chairs were upset. It certainly looked as if there had been a fight here.

The husband had various injuries:
- A superficial incision of his upper chest.
- A wound that penetrated three centimetres into his left, lower leg.
- Two slightly deeper, small injuries on the palm of his right hand.
- A stab wound to the heart that had penetrated the anterior wall of the right ventricle and left a smaller injury at the apex.

He had been rushed to hospital and extensive heart surgery had been attempted, so there was a lot of suturing. The surgery was eventually unsuccessful and, of course, it was this wound to the heart that had proved fatal.

However, at a superficial glance, his injuries did not look as bad as his wife's. I did not meet her or examine her myself; instead I reviewed the many photos taken of her wounds. I was looking for self-inflicted injuries, the sign of a murderer who plans to plead self-defence.

Pathologists frequently have to decide between homicide and suicide, accidental and deliberate injuries. And knife wounds are the realm of the faker: they look so horrible that at first glance the inexperienced must immediately believe that no one could possibly do that to themselves. I have learned over the years, however, that there is almost nothing people will not do to avoid a murder charge. Self-inflicted injuries are generally recognizable: they are created with the minimum force to create maximum effect, and obviously they are always in parts of the body which are readily accessible to its owner's hand. Injuries which cannot possibly be self-inflicted are also identifiable, and, because of this, I am sometimes pleased to help relieve the innocent of assault charges.

The wife in this case had:
- Bruising to her left upper arm, left shoulder, left side of neck, right hip, left hip, right thigh, right hand.
- A gaping incised wound, but not a deep wound, on the front left side of the neck.
- Superficial scratches in the same area.
- A puncture wound by the neck wound.
- An incision over the collar bone.
- Incisions on the back of the left elbow.
- A horizontal incision under the right breast.
- Short stab wounds on both sides of the abdomen.
- A puncture wound in the right thigh.

- A gaping incision on the right hand.
- Short, superficial cuts on the right thumb.
- A knife graze on the left hand.
- A broken tooth.

The Crown Prosecution Service had many meetings about this case. When the late husband's family picked up the possibility that the wife might not be charged, they furiously talked of a civil prosecution. They hired Iain to write a report comparing the description of the fight the wife had given the police with her actual wounds.

And here was his report, waiting on my desk when I returned from Manchester. It was so thunderous that it was practically rumbling.

The blunt injuries to the arm could have resulted from a series of blows to the arm. The pattern does not appear to be typical of gripping . . .

While it is possible for individuals to produce bruises on their own body by striking themselves with objects or by pinching etc., in this instance the injuries on the arm could be the result of an assault by the husband.

The overall pattern of her injuries, however, is not at all typical of the type of wounds which would have been sustained if there had been a vigorous assault by the deceased who had been attempting to stab her. Skin is one of the toughest tissues in the body and once the tip of a knife has pierced skin, assuming even a moderate degree of force behind the thrust, there would be nothing to stop the instrument from penetrating deeply into the body: in many instances the blade penetrates to full length. All of the wounds seen on this lady's body appear to be very superficial and there does not appear to be any substantial degree of penetration.

Self-inflicted, incised wounds in the neck are not uncommon. There is no evidence to suggest that the knife had been thrust into the neck in a stabbing motion. Given the manner in which the wounds were alleged to have been caused on her abdomen, I am firmly of the opinion that they are not consistent with deliberate forceful knife thrusts but are consistent with self-injury or stab injuries inflicted under considerable control.

This lady may have been the victim of an assault involving blows such as punches or even blows from a chair, although I can see little evidence to sustain an allegation of heavy kicks to the thighs or of the head being forcibly struck against the floor. The overall pattern of the wounds is, however, consistent with self-injury.

I agreed that the wife had been subjected to a blunt trauma attack. I disagreed that the knife wounds were self-inflicted.

I gave several reasons for this.

First, when she was stabbed in the abdomen she had described this as feeling like punches, not like being cut or stabbed at all. This is a very common misperception of an individual who is stabbed: time and time again I have heard victims say that they could just feel a punch rather than the knife itself penetrating. This is a fact, but it is not the kind of fact that the wife is likely to have known.

Second, although she could have injured her own neck and abdomen, it would be very difficult and most unusual for someone to injure the back of one elbow and the back of the opposite hand.

Third, it was the husband's injuries that were most important and, of his four stab or incised injuries, three were in non-lethal areas of the body. The unusual stab wound to the leg did suggest that his wife was on the floor when it was inflicted, or anyway she was low down. The fatal wound to the heart may have been inflicted deliberately, but in the context of a struggle for control of the knife I felt that it was not possible to exclude *beyond reasonable doubt* the possibility that the wound was inflicted accidentally. And no one could maintain, from the blunt trauma injuries on the wife, that there had not been a very serious struggle.

So, although the case was full of doubts and discrepancies, as an expert witness I couldn't state beyond reasonable doubt that the fatal stab wound to the husband was deliberate or that the wounds to the wife were self-inflicted. Even on the lower level of guilt, the balance of probabilities, I felt that it was the husband and not the wife who had inflicted her wounds.

The Crown Prosecution Service decided that it would not be in the interests of the public – or the public purse – to pursue this case. The coroner, aware that a very angry family was sitting in his court, ensured the police were present for the inquest. Iain did not give his statement in person, although, of course, there was reference to it. My evidence was punctuated by angry cries and much scoffing. The coroner more than once had to call for calm.

My opinion was vindicated when the coroner gave the verdict of justifiable homicide. It was delivered to a court which, for a moment, listened in complete silence. And then broke into uproar.

I slipped away as the shouting worsened. So far as I am aware, the threatened civil action against the wife did not materialize. When I got home, Chris was out and Anna was bending over her physics books in a bubble of concentration. She reminded me of Jen. As I carried in the thick files from the knifing case, I wondered if I had ever pored over my books with such concentration or if, like Chris, I had been more erratic.

'What have you been doing today?' she asked.

I told her about the coroner's court, the angry relatives. It was the first time she had ever inquired directly about my job.

To my amazement, she said, 'Can I see the photos?'

The one thing she did know about my work was that the pictures were taboo.

'The photos of . . . ?'

'The husband's body.'

She was fifteen and studying for her GCSEs. I shook my head. 'You're a bit young to look at pictures from the mortuary.'

'No, really, I want to see them. I've seen loads of diagrams in biology.'

'But your biology book diagrams don't have stab wounds.'

'I really think I can take it, Dad.'

Maybe she was right. Maybe it was time to stop shielding my children from the unusual nature of my work. Maybe all those fixed specimens in my study that were en route to lectures or court (it was scarcely possible to hide them all), the medical talk at mealtimes, maybe it all meant death was more routine for her than I'd realized.

I said, 'I'll show you the wounds on the wife and we'll see how you get on. Since she's very much alive. And you can tell me if you think she stabbed herself to make it look as if her husband attacked her.'

Anna's eyes lit up.

'I thought she didn't, the coroner thought she didn't, but Iain West wrote a scathing report saying she did.'

Anna nodded enthusiastically.

'And this is not, I repeat not, to be discussed with anyone outside this family,' I added sternly. She gave me a withering look.

'Duh. I know all that.'

We spent an odd but strangely bonding half hour discussing wounds. Their ugliness seemed not to bother Anna at all. Finally, at her pleading, I showed her the pictures of the husband, of the stab wound to the heart that had killed him. Cleaned up in the mortuary, it looked unspectacular.

'He's just like an asleep person,' she said. 'Dead bodies aren't scary really.'

'They aren't scary at all, but I'm not showing you the pictures of his insides, all the same.'

She shrugged.

'OK,' she said, 'but it wouldn't bother me.'

It did occur to me, for the first time, that Anna might be discovering her inner pathologist.

'I thought you and Chris both wanted to be vets,' I said.

'He does. I do. But I might want to be a doctor.'

'Well, I wouldn't think of becoming a pathologist, certainly not a forensic pathologist.'

She blinked at me in surprise. Even I was surprised to hear myself.

'But Mum says you love your job!' she protested.

'I do. But . . .' But what? Suddenly the courtroom humiliations, the angry relatives, the many faces of grief, the healthy old ladies whose deaths no one had thought suspicious and who had now been disturbed in their graves: it all seemed like something I wanted my daughter to avoid.

'Dad?' She sounded alarmed. 'What's up?'

I said, 'Anna, I've just realized something. It's time I took up flying again.'

## 30

The inquiry Stephen Lawrence's family had fought so hard for was finally drawing to a close with the century. In his final report, early in 1999, Sir William Macpherson said, 'We believe that the immediate impact of the inquiry . . . has brought forcibly before the public the justifiable complaints of Mr and Mrs Lawrence, and the hitherto underplayed dissatisfaction and unhappiness of minority ethnic communities, both locally and all over the country, in connection with this and other cases, as to their treatment by police.'

The police's investigation into Stephen Lawrence's death was described as 'palpably flawed' and I believe it was here that the public first encountered the expression 'institutional racism'. The inquiry and its revelations marked a significant change in the public's attitude to the police: they were no longer necessarily the trustworthy friends of the innocent. And, within the Met, perhaps the inquiry also led to the beginning of a change in attitudes towards minority communities.

For the Lawrence family, it was not all over yet. The rest of their story is well known: it unfolded over the next thirteen years and perhaps continues to unfold. At least partly due to this case, in 2005 the double jeopardy law was revised, with the result that the accused can now sometimes be retried for the same crime if new evidence has been found. By 2011, scientific advances had found Stephen's DNA on the suspects' clothing and this was sufficient new evidence to put the suspects on trial again. It was my most recent, although perhaps not my last, court appearance for this case. In January 2012, Gary Dobson and David Norris were found guilty of murder and given life sentences of approximately fourteen years each. Three of Stephen's murderers remained at large, at least for that crime. The main suspects have been openly named many times.

Back to the end of the 1990s, where life at St George's felt deceptively stable and life in general was elevated by flight. Because I could now fly solo. Yes, one cold, clear January day, I went up there. Into the sky. Completely alone.

I do not know why having nothing but air beneath me, above me, on all sides of me, offered such a release from my job's harsh realities. I do not know why being surrounded by so much space and having the means to navigate through it gave me an illusion of control over my own destiny that nothing fixed to the earth could offer. I do not know why sitting at the controls of a small aircraft simply wiped out the complications that kept my brain whirring in circles so much of the time. I just know that I loved it, and all the time I flew I thought about nothing but now, nothing but flying the plane.

I began to look forward to the time when flying would not be confined to Friday afternoons with the Met. This year Anna would take GCSEs and Chris A-levels. Our home lives, and to some extent our working lives, had always revolved around our children. They didn't need someone there all the time now, although they needed support in a different way. But in a few years, they would both be gone. It was a certainty, a horrible one. We would have to rethink our world. And acknowledge that a day would come when our work would be done.

That was why we bought a cottage on the Isle of Man. We had fallen in love with it one holiday. It was not far from Austin and Maggie's house and it would need a lot of work but we had agreed that, eventually, we would like to live there all the time. Although eventually seemed far, far away.

In 1999 I finally did stop smoking. New millennium, new century, did I really want to welcome it in through a haze of lung-congesting cigarette smoke? No, I did not. Did I really want to limit my chances of seeing more than a few years of the century by consuming industrial quantities of expensive carcinogens on a daily basis? No, I did not. And, although I had tried many times before to give up, it was the impending arrival of the year 2000 which meant that this time I was successful. After four or five months of grumpiness, nicotine gum and jaws like a hamster from chewing it, I reached a sweet point. I suddenly knew I could live without cigarettes and that I would go into the new century without ever smoking again. And I haven't.

We saw in the New Year on the Isle of Man.

'I do want to live here,' said Jen. 'That's what I really want for the next century.'

'I think I'll have my pilot's licence soon. We could live here and just fly everywhere we need to go,' I said. Places are always nicer when you fly to them. But I was in no rush. I wasn't fifty yet and the Isle of Man was a retire-ment sort of place. Wasn't it?

Chris was planning to start vet's training in the next year or two. Anna was studying for A-levels and still agoniz-ing between becoming a vet and a doctor.

'Dad, I think it would be a very good idea if I came to a post-mortem,' she said one day.

Reflex reaction: no.

Anna, so young, so inexperienced, with her smooth cheeks and bright eyes, should not be confronted by life's ugly realities in the mortuary, that was obvious.

'Chris went! And he wasn't even sixteen!'

'Chris was simply shown through the post-mortem room by an idiot coroner's officer. And he wasn't very happy about it.'

'This would be different, because I'd be prepared. You'd talk me through it, wouldn't you?'

No.

'And when I apply to medical school, think how it would look on my personal statement. I bet no one else applying will have watched a post-mortem.'

No.

So she came with me to a mortuary one day. Not to see a victim of suicide or homicide but a few sudden, natural deaths. As we leaned over the body, I glanced up at Anna, her brows knitted with concentration, as I pointed out that brain haemorrhage, that entirely occluded coronary artery, that cirrhotic liver, which looked so like a mottled mackerel.

'If you go into medicine, you don't have to become a

pathologist,' I reminded her on the way home. 'Talk to your mother about dermatology.'

She said, 'I have. I just wonder if I'm not more of a pathologist, really.'

It was strange to think of the next generation of Shepherds being grown-up and out there working. Because that meant the last generation must be getting old.

I knew this for sure one summer day in 2001 when I found myself attending the funeral of Iain West. He had died, aged only fifty-seven, of lung cancer, caused, I can say without doubt, by his smoking – a habit that, of course, I had shared until recently.

We had known he was dying for a few months, but when I heard the news, I could hardly believe it. I had seen him not long ago at Westminster coroner's court. He had come to give evidence: nothing could keep the old trooper away. Perhaps he knew it would be the last time he'd take the oath and hold a court in thrall. Downstairs, in the offices, I thought how much he had aged and how diminished he looked. He climbed the stairs to the oak-panelled courtroom very slowly – but no one dared to offer assistance. Then when he rose to give evidence and took the oath, there was a metamorphosis. The old Iain West was still there. Still in command. Still a presence.

Now that he was gone I felt keenly that, as well as being my mentor and teacher, my opponent and rival, he had also been my friend. Those long conferences in his office and in the pub, the sudden kindnesses, the knowing but unacknowledged intimacy of colleagues who have worked closely together for many years – it was no less a friendship for being office-based. And now my friend simply was not there any more and I had not made enough effort to see him and enjoy his company during his last illness and enforced semi-retirement.

As if this was not melancholy enough, there was double devastation because, on that same day, Jen's father, the estimable Austin, died on the Isle of Man, leaving the family heartbroken.

Not one memento mori, but two. You might think that, since we constantly stare death in the face, pathologists don't need to be reminded of our own mortality. We do. We, too, need prompting by the death of those close to us to get on with the things we want to do in life. For Jen and me, living on the lovely Isle of Man was one of those things. Now we wondered if we shouldn't do it sooner rather than later. We also thought Jen's mother, the widowed Maggie, might need us. It was time seriously to recognize that, if we wanted to live on the island, this was not something we could put off for ever.

That year, 2001, also saw the release of the final reports on the *Marchioness* disaster. Lord Justice Clarke held both a formal inquiry into the disaster itself and a non-statutory inquiry (which is more flexible and generally regarded as less 'clunking' in its approach) into the handling of the *Marchioness* dead and their relatives. After the formal inquiry, there were still more recommendations for the improvement of safety and lifeguarding systems on the Thames. And, at the non-statutory inquiry, Lord Justice Clarke confirmed that the *Marchioness* relatives were the victims of a human and systems failure. His report recognized the muddles in management and identification procedures: he noted confusions between key figures who were on holiday and their deputies, between the many ranks of police officers, between police, coroner and fingerprint officers, between coroner's officers, between the mortuary staff and the undertakers.

As for me, the inquiry closed a chapter of my life. The pathologists were at last exonerated of any blame for the errors that had been made. Eleven years after the disaster I was finally free of the fury the identification problems, particularly the missing hands, had generated. The angry phone calls and press disdain that had reappeared periodically in my life for so long, stopped overnight.

The non-statutory inquiry report's wider interest was its many recommendations for the treatment of relatives and the identification of victims in a disaster. It happened that for a few years now I had myself been giving quite a bit of thought to this problem. During the 1990s I had been asking myself how well we – forensic pathologists and crisis teams in general – would cope in London with a mass disaster. Because disasters were changing.

By 2001 our transport systems and cities were much safer than in the past. The greatest threat now was terrorism. IRA bombings of the 1970s and 80s and into the 90s were still in our consciousness. And other cities had suffered. In 1993 a bomb exploded at the World Trade Center in New York, killing six people and injuring over a hundred. In 1995 cultists gassed the Tokyo subway with Sarin.

The coroner for West London, Alison Thompson, shared my concern about planning – or rather the lack of it – for both natural and unnatural disasters. Her jurisdiction covered the Fulham mortuary where St George's pathologists worked but, more significantly, Heathrow airport. In the event of a mass disaster in London there was an existing understanding that bodies would be brought to a special hangar at the airport. We decided to go and have a look at it. And found something that was more like a large garage. It was full of runway snow-ploughs and ancillary equipment.

It would have been hard to find a site less suitable. Apart from the fact that it was dirty and oily and full of heavy plant, access was difficult and there was only one small hand basin. We proposed to the police, the other emergency services, local authorities and the supporting charities that we should all review London's plans for a large-scale emergency. It turned out that we weren't alone in worrying about how the capital would cope in such an event and everyone was keen to participate.

We knew how to define an emergency. Dr David Paul, the retired coroner for North London, had once done so very simply, saying, 'My idea of an emergency is having at least one more body than my mortuary can manage.'

Our group met regularly at Heathrow Police Station and the first thing we did was try to anticipate what sort of emergencies might occur. We frequently sat around tables drinking coffee and discussing how to deal with a flu pandemic. Or a big plane crash in the city. Or a terrorist attack. But we knew that, no matter how bizarre and outrageous our thoughts, the reality would always be different and that we needed to think and plan from the specific to the general.

And we were proved correct. Chris was just about to leave home. His bags were packed and he was soon to catch a train north to study veterinary science when he phoned me.

'Anna and I are watching it on TV . . .'

'Watching what?'

'Dad, are you on call for international emergencies?'

That day was 11 September 2001.

I switched on the TV and stared at footage of American Airlines Flight 11 hitting the North Tower of the World Trade Center. This at first looked like the kind of terrible accident our group had talked about. But when United Airlines Flight 175 hit the South Tower shortly afterwards, I realized that, although we had discussed both acts of terrorism and city plane crashes, it had never occurred to us that the two would be combined in such a deadly way.

Then, incredibly, impossibly, as the world watched, the Twin Towers actually fell. First the South. And then the North. And now it seemed to me that these terrorists had taken disaster to a level that was far, far beyond anything we could have dreamed of.

I was as appalled and mesmerized as the rest of the world by this spectacular coup. The possibility of my own involvement did not occur to me. I assumed my colleagues in America would get on with the massive job of saving the wounded and finding and identifying the dead: what was there for the British to contribute? But Alison Thompson was soon on the phone.

As the coroner for West London, Alison would be receiving any repatriated British bodies at Heathrow and it would be her job to establish a cause of death. Any British citizen who dies abroad is entitled to an inquest in the

UK by law: this has been the case since 1982, when the father of a young British nurse who died in sleazy circumstances in Saudi Arabia refused to accept the official cause given for her death, and the consequent change in the law has resonated through the decades.

Alison was also well aware that, when a civilian plane had been downed by a terrorist bomb over Lockerbie in Scotland more than ten years earlier, a number of mistakes had been made in the management, not least the identification, of just a few of the bodies. But 'a few' mistakes in this critical situation has the effect of destabilizing and distressing a huge number of families.

Alison's concerns about the management of the British fatalities resulted in the rapid formation of a group at Scotland Yard consisting not only of the police and emergency services members of our existing mass disaster committee, but also many more high-ranking officials.

The questions we asked were: What support can we offer the New York operation? How should we repatriate our dead? Should we carry out our own post-mortems on the British fatalities back here in the UK? Would the families find acceptable that further interference with the bodies of their loved ones? Or should we leave all post-mortems and identifications to the Office of the Chief Medical Examiner (OCME) of New York? If we repatriated the bodies, they could be distributed around the country to their own local coroners, in which case should each local coroner hold an inquest and reach his or her own verdict? We could imagine inquests going on for months or even years and there would probably, certainly, be a huge range of different and maybe conflicting verdicts, ranging from accidental death to homicide to unlawful killing.

We agreed we should assess what OCME in New York was doing first. We could then determine a formal UK response and offer appropriate help.

We reported directly to the prime minister, Tony Blair, at the Cabinet Office's central emergency co-ordinating group, COBRA. They decided we needed some first-hand opinions and so it was finally determined that on 20 September – the day on which I became forty-nine years old – I would fly out to New York to see how the Americans at the Office of the Chief Medical Examiner were handling things. I phoned my colleague at OCME, Yvonne Milewski, and arranged to meet her on my arrival. She sounded tired and emotionally drained. But welcoming all the same.

I landed in a New York that was strangely quiet, even for the middle of the night. The city was still hushed with horror. Nine days after the towers had collapsed, the event's dust and smell still hung in the air. And although roads were blocked and tunnels were closed, when the traffic stood still not one horn honked. I told the taxi driver where I was staying and he said there were at least four hotels of that name. So we drove through quiet streets trying them all. Eventually we knew we'd found the right one because the lobby was full of British police officers, some of whom I recognized. They gave me a warm welcome and asked me if I fancied a drink, but I had to decline. I'd arranged to meet Yvonne at the OCME mortuary and was taking a cab straight there.

I arrived at 2.30 in the morning to an unforgettable

sight. The building itself was an ugly 1960s concrete pill box, but the building was not the focus of attention. The surrounding streets and parking lots had been partitioned off and were fully guarded because here was the twenty-four-hour receiving area. Once through security I was into a makeshift, floodlit resting plaza, full of tented cafes and workers taking a break over coffee and doughnuts. Beyond were huge, refrigerated trailers, at least thirty of them, lined up neatly in adjacent tented parking lots, flowers guarding the entrances, American flags standing sadly sentinel.

I sniffed. That aroma. It was obvious the trailers were full of human body parts.

Even at this time of night, an occasional hearse reversed into the docking bay with a body bag on board. The search crews at Ground Zero were working around the clock and the pathologists were working too: Yvonne had volunteered for the night shift. And the day shift. She just grabbed sleep when she could.

You needed huge resilience to cope in this bizarre and disturbing environment. Many people found that they didn't actually have that resilience and the mental trauma to the rescue workers and to the mortuary staff was huge. Some coped. Some were sent home, looking like people with shellshock.

The shift pattern meant that there was never a delay in the start of the formal examination and identification process. Some of the body bags were known to contain a member of the police or fire service who had risked – and lost – his or her life in the carnage. For these Members of Service, a colour party formed which formally saluted their bravery as they were carried in to OCME.

Inside the many body bags were whole, or almost whole, bodies. Smaller body parts sometimes came in smaller boxes. The basic rule of all disaster recovery sites is that if a rescue worker finds, say, a finger, even if it seems quite clear which body that finger belongs to, it must be catalogued separately and given a unique number. The nature of this disaster, the huge forces from the impacts and from the collapses, meant that the bodies were frequently so fragmented that you simply couldn't put people together by sight, guided by their location or clothes. It was clear, very early on, that many or maybe most of the identifications would have to rely on DNA. Later, sometimes much later, based on this amazing technique, limbs, portions, parts, pieces and fragments of tissue would come together to reform something like a body, or what remained of it. As in all mass disasters, identification of the victims was to be a huge administrative as well as scientific operation. It was just that in this disaster the task was in every way bigger, worse and harder than anything experienced before.

As they arrived, bodies were taken into the primary receiving room where preliminary examinations were performed. And then they were taken directly to one of the examination suites. Each suite had a full team of police, pathologists, photographers, radiologists and assistants. Post-mortems were carried out in the usual way, on whole bodies or parts of bodies. Extensive details were recorded and these findings were linked with the fragments of clothing, personal artefacts – jewellery, credit cards, etc. – and any other features and details of where exactly the body had been found. Then, carefully numbered, the body or body part was taken to its unique place on a uniquely numbered shelf inside a uniquely numbered trailer.

The bodies were treated with great respect and the trailers were kept clean and well ordered, the Stars and Stripes a reminder of the state and the containers of flowers a reminder of the people. The trailers solved the key problem of any such disaster: not so much processing the dead as storing them until the identification can be made. After that, they can be released to the families. It was clear to me that the Americans were doing a fantastic job of looking after things, methodically and respectfully.

I tried to remain as unobtrusive as possible, since everyone on site was working hard. The same was true when I returned the next day to meet the chief medical examiner himself, Charles Hirsch. He was a small, slight and distinctly stressed man in his mid-sixties who was running this massive operation with stitches across his head and some fractured ribs. He had been among the early rescue workers who arrived at the World Trade Center just before the first of the towers fell. How had he escaped with comparatively minor injuries when the colleagues who had been standing next to him were felled by rubble and were now in intensive care?

The trailers were filling fast. Eventually it was concluded that there were 2,753 victims, and in total something like 70,000 body parts or fragments were found. Many of the bodies had been pulverized, either by the initial explosion or when the buildings came down. It would have been a lot easier to have put everything into one mass grave but, of course, the families of the dead could not bear the idea that their loved ones might be buried with the hijackers.

Soon, all the rubble from the World Trade Center was being shifted to an old landfill site on Staten Island in the Hudson Bay Estuary, strangely called Fresh Kills. It was sifted, every bit of it, not once but twice by a skilled team led by police and the FBI, which included anthropologists and doctors. And then the long journey through the DNA of almost 3,000 people began. Each tiny fragment of human tissue, each personal effect had to be identified.

This programme in fact continued for many years: identifications were still being made in 2013. Finally, in 2015, 1,637 victims had been identified, accounting for just 60 per cent of those believed to have died: the others had become dust, as all bodies must. Now there are plans to turn Fresh Kills into one of the world's largest urban parks.

An anthropologist friend who worked sifting through the debris was, like many others involved in the disaster, traumatized by it. After months of sieving for bits of human tissue and bone she developed a horror of flying. When she returned to the UK, before boarding her flight she wrote her name on every part of her body, every single limb, in case the plane crashed and she was dismembered. In fact, it was many years before she worked again.

Towards the end of my brief trip, I was driven to a nondescript building in Manhattan that was one of the British Consulate offices in New York. A Foreign Office team from the UK was waiting for me. At that time, we knew there were many British dead but not how many.

'So,' demanded one of the officials, 'how are we going to get our British bodies home?'

I wondered how they imagined the repatriation of the bodies to be. Then one of them, a politician, talked about a row of coffins being driven in slow convoy from the airport to London, each draped in the British flag.

I shook my head. I had been up for almost two days and I was shocked and tired. From the coalface, this line of flag-decked hearses sounded like a politically motivated stunt to maximize the drama and photo opportunity for the government. I felt something dangerous rising inside me, something really terrifying, something that, if I had let it, could have turned into fury. And I am never angry, let alone furious. But now something escaped.

'Coffins? Did you say coffins? Most of these people have been pulverized, don't you understand that? Instead of coffins you'll probably be sending them back in matchboxes!'

They glared back at me. There was little further dialogue. I was thanked and dismissed.

My report praised the Americans' handling of the disaster, saying that we could use their paperwork instead of creating our own. As a result, although the final death toll for Britain was, in fact, sixty-seven, just one coroner's court in the UK, run by an experienced and empathic coroner, dealt with every British fatality. Just one American police officer flew over to give evidence. And there was just one verdict. It was unlawful killing.

*

Four years later, London too came under Islamist attack. On 7 July 2005, fifty-two people were killed and more than 700 injured when four terrorist bombs exploded, three of them on the London Underground and one on a bus. Literally a few days earlier, with the involvement now of many agencies, the mass-disaster plan that the coroner Alison Thompson and I had started thinking about back in the 1990s had been signed off.

I was not in London at the time but when the appeal went up for help I flew straight back and set to work in the excellent, tented temporary mortuary facility that had been constructed in less than forty-eight hours on the playing field at the Honourable Artillery Company in the City. All the bodies were taken here and the facility, indeed our whole plan, proved fully functional. I carried out my work with immense sorrow. Perhaps, deep down, in some irrational place, I might have hoped that, by making a plan, we would be saved from ever putting it into action. What wishful thinking.

The coroners in charge of that crisis may have had one regret. Relatives of *Marchioness* victims had bitterly criticized the need for the full post-mortems we had carried out, saying they were unnecessary since the cause of death after such a disaster was clear. Consequently, after the 2005 bombings we were told not to carry out full post-mortems. Our job was identification only. If we opened bodies, it was purely to look for the gall bladder and appendix because if they had been removed this might assist identification.

Afterwards, extraordinarily, the ambulance service was criticized for being too slow in recovering the wounded.

Crews do not go where they may be harmed and, because there was a risk that further bombs had been planted, they had been told to wait before entering the bomb sites. Accusations followed that this delay had actually been responsible for a number of deaths. There was a suggestion that lawyers for some victims' families would seek compensation from the emergency services. Because full post-mortems had not been carried out, we pathologists struggled to answer the questions asked by both families and the coroner to resolve these claims.

I did learn from this. Years later, I was the pathologist in charge when taxi driver Derrick Bird went on a killing spree in Cumbria. It was highly reminiscent of Michael Ryan's massacre in Hungerford more than twenty years earlier. Some people pressed me not to perform full post-mortems on the grounds that it was obvious what the cause of death was. Mindful of 7/7, I did not give in to their entreaties. Every patient first had an MRI scan to reveal the position of every bullet, and each body was given a full post-mortem. There was not one criticism of the emergency services' response.

## 31

My second brush with the work of Osama bin Laden was in Bali a year after 9/11. Two bombs planted by Islamic extremists connected to bin Laden exploded in crowded tourist areas of this lovely Indonesian island and more than 200 were killed, most of them Western holidaymakers and most of them under thirty.

Once again, at a few hours' notice I found myself on a plane. I was sitting next to some rather bulky men. I thought possibly they were from special forces. In fact, we didn't speak the whole way, although I guessed that we were all flying east for the same reason. I assumed they thought I was a tourist or a reporter. However, when there was no one to meet me at Denpasar Airport, they noticed this and turned to me by the luggage carousel for the first time.

'Want a lift, Doc?'

'How did you know who I am?'

'We guessed you must be the pathologist just by looking at you.'

'How?'

'Well, for a start you didn't laugh at the movie.'

That's pathologists for you. Miserable, death-obsessed, dour-faced butchers. But I was grateful for the lift. And the first person I saw at the hotel was coroner Alison Thompson, who happened to have been staying in Hong Kong and had flown directly here, knowing, again, that the British bodies would fall under her jurisdiction when they arrived at Heathrow. We greeted each other warmly and, although it was early morning in Bali, decided to set off for the hospital where the bodies were being stored.

Before leaving London, I had been told that I was simply viewing the operation from the British point of view. But when I walked into the mortuary the other pathologists (mostly Australians but also Dutch and Germans) recognized me from international meetings we'd all attended and immediately handed me a gown, an apron, some rubber gloves and a knife. And said, 'Get on with it, Dick.'

The British embassy staff had done an amazing job of locating the British bodies. Not only that, they had found the fuel to keep the generator going of one of the few chilled containers in the whole place – if not the whole country. In fact, as with all disasters, we pathologists just worked a conveyor-belt system of post-mortems, taking whichever body came next, whatever the nationality.

The problem was lack of facilities for the dead in a world of intense heat. I will never forget the sight or the smell of the bodies laid out in the shade, covered with bags of ice cubes from the supermarket. How I longed to find a lorry full of ice which we could tip all over them. They were changing fast, and not for the better. Many were already fragmented and identification was the usual jigsaw challenge, only made more complex by the untrained recovery teams who just threw everything they found in one area into one bag. It was a great relief to come across an isolated hand wearing a wedding ring which was engraved on the inside with the name of its bearer. It was a small, tragic item and it gave us one small piece of the tragic puzzle.

Most of the victims who had been attracted to that sybaritic island were young and beautiful. They had been enjoying themselves in the bar or nightclub where the two bombs exploded, one after the other. The bombs were planted by an extremist group believed to be funded by al-Qaeda.

Eventually it was confirmed that there were twenty-eight British fatalities and that overall more than 200 people were injured and 202 were killed. It was a hard, exhausting and traumatic time. I have subsequently visited the memorials to this atrocity both in London and in Perth, Western Australia, but no memorial is necessary to remind me of the decaying bodies, the ice, the smell, the single dripping tap in the mortuary that was our water supply and the overarching sense of the futility of terrorism. I am not sure it has ever really left me.

Back home, my working life was feeling insecure. The world of forensic pathology was changing and we were now threatened by new uncertainties of a sort the great Simpson never had to face. The university medical schools had always paid us to lecture in our subject but they decided – almost all of them, one by one – that now they would not continue funding or teaching forensic pathology. The main reason they gave was lack of forensic research and lack of publication in prestigious scientific journals. However, we were too busy with post-mortems and coroners and courts to meet these new benchmarks of a Good University. The age of intellectual evaluation through research assessment exercise had arrived. And we forensic pathologists were found wanting.

Gradually, medical schools with great traditions of forensic pathology closed down departments and it wasn't long after Iain West's death that his kingdom at Guy's disappeared. St George's hung on a bit longer, but my new department's warrant for execution had been signed.

We had essentially been privatized. From now on, instead of providing forensic services for free, our salaries paid by the universities at which we taught, we would directly bill the police, coroners or defence solicitors for payment.

I knew that, without a salary, it would be hard to continue with some necessary but unpaid work. I am talking about public work, like my ongoing contribution to teaching the authorities safe restraint methods. And my participation in disaster planning. Everyone else at the group was salaried by the police or some other organization: I no longer had the weight of a university behind me.

Not only was the regular income gone, so were lectures and so were students, except at just a few specialist centres outside London. I had only ever lectured to packed halls and knew how interesting medical students found forensic work. I also felt that at least the rudiments of forensic medicine should be an important part of their training. Every doctor, no matter what their discipline, should be able to identify the signs of suspicious circumstances so that they would know when to call an expert or the police. But there was too much 'real' medicine competing for too little space in the training schedules and forensic pathology now became accessible only on specialist post-graduate courses at few universities.

I set up a group called Forensic Pathology Services, widely known as FPS, through which pathologists in London and the south-east of the UK would operate in our brave new privatized world. And suddenly, while I was buried deep in its planning and organization, I realized that I might not want to be a part of it.

With a heavy heart, I had dropped Anna off that autumn at university: she had finally decided to study medicine. So they were gone now, both of our children, to the north of England. Of course, they still needed us, but not in the same way. Our house seemed large and empty and quiet. Was that why we were spending more and more time on the Isle of Man? That home was nearer the children than London. Was it because, as my lectureship duties at St George's were being wound down, there was little to keep us here? Was it because we loved our cottage on the island and wanted to support Jen's now-widowed mother – not that Maggie had let widowhood stand in the way of her social life – and in fact were now ourselves becoming part of her whirl?

Or . . . was my work in London beginning to weary me? Weary me so much that even flying on Friday afternoons could not restore me? Every court appearance seemed to turn into a bruising scrap and sometimes I felt I lacked the resilience to cope with it. There was no longer a bounce in my step when the police called me to another crime, another body. I had given up hope that they would ever phone me for my opinion on a case. And, looking into the future, I could see that pathologists eventually could be tendering for contracts, competing for bodies, even undercutting each other on price. Forensic pathology was a service, but no longer the intellectually rigorous world I had entered, with its scope for debate, study and social change.

Jen had become disillusioned with her work, too. Despite her amazing feat in becoming a doctor so late in life, once she was practising as a GP she found she did not really want to be one. She had always been keen for us to move to the Isle of Man and believed that here she could practise her own specialization, dermatology, and live in the place she wanted to be.

What else pushed us there? Our knowledge of our own senescence? A longing for the lifestyle Maggie and Austin had enjoyed? A hope that, if we spent more time isolated together on an island, somehow the loving communication which was missing would suddenly reappear?

Perhaps I – and perhaps Jen too – was having that thing people call a mid-life crisis, which no pathologist has ever been able to locate within the human body, not even under a microscope. But when I was asked to write the twelfth edition of *Simpson's Forensic Medicine* (the third edition of which you may remember had lured me into this profession), the invitation felt like a huge honour. And an excuse. So I was midwife to, but did not remain with, the new Forensic Pathology Services. Instead, Jen and I left London for good. We gave up the tidy hedges and neatly mown lawns of Surrey for a windswept and beautiful cottage on an island somewhere off Liverpool. I was generally believed, by my colleagues and contemporaries, to have completely lost my marbles.

I was very happy and busy renovating the cottage. We went walking for miles over wild and windy moorland under big, big skies that were sometimes so clear we could see across the water to where the Mountains of Mourne sweep down to the sea. We sat by the fire while gales whistled outside. Or we just stared across the fields to the ocean as it conjured up dramatic storms from its depths. I did not carry out a single post-mortem.

And, here we had a social life. We had always been too busy for this before but now we had friends. It mattered little that we were much younger than most of them. We simply slotted into the society that had been ready-made for us by Maggie. So what if she was ageing a little now? She was still at every party, a woman with haute couture dresses bulging from every wardrobe in almost every bedroom in the house. Something delicious bubbling on the stove, a gin and tonic always at the ready and she was never without an admiring circle of friends. It felt good to be among them, good to be part of a community. The children visited often.

For me there may have been no more post-mortems, but there was lots of interesting work. I was writing my text-book on forensic pathology. I flew myself to the mainland to sit on committees for the British Association in Forensic Medicine, who were still sorting out Home Office contracts and many other details of the new privatized landscape. I was asked to give opinions on complex cases. I was busy on several ministerial working groups, devising and promoting more humane methods of restraint.

Of course, I kept an eye on all interesting developments in my field. I learned that the police had reopened the inquiry into Rachel Nickell's murder: they now, finally, began to accept that someone other than Colin Stagg might have killed her. It took another six years for developments in DNA testing to nail Robert Napper for her death, the man who had murdered Samantha Bisset so violently and who was already detained in Broadmoor for life. I recalled carrying out the second post-mortem on Samantha Bisset's mutilated body and I remembered saying to the detective how much I was reminded of Rachel Nickell's murder. I wished now that I hadn't simply made a passing remark but said something more forceful, more questioning, more insistent.

There was also a major development in the case of Sally Clark, the mother convicted of killing her two baby sons. She seemed to be planning a second appeal. She had been in jail for over two years now, but this appeal would be based on new evidence. New pathological evidence.

The results of tests performed on blood and tissue samples taken from her second child had been discovered. The pathologist had not revealed this evidence before. In the view of some experts, but certainly not all, it showed that the second child might have died naturally of a bacterial (staphylococcal) infection.

The Court of Appeal's job was to assess whether, if the jury had been in possession of this information at the time of the trial, it might reasonably have affected their decision to convict. The three judges decided that it might, and that therefore the conviction was unsafe.

In 2003 Sally Clark, by that time a broken alcoholic, was released from jail. She died four years later.

Sir Roy Meadow, the man who produced the extraordinary statistic that there was a 1 in 73 million chance of two children from the same family dying naturally, was publicly discredited. A number of the other mothers he had given evidence against and who were serving sentences now launched successful appeals. His maths was challenged by statisticians and he was struck off by the General Medical Council. He later, much later, won his appeal against being struck off, but by then he was over seventy. One piece of bad, off-the-cuff, maths in court under intense cross-examination was a sad ending to a previously highly distinguished career.

The pathologist, he who had examined both babies, changed his cause of death in one of them and apparently withheld test results, was found guilty by the GMC of serious misconduct. He was suspended from carrying out Home Office post-mortems for eighteen months.

David Southall had been a commentator on, rather than a direct participant in, the Clark brothers' case but Sally Clark's release now catalysed the inevitable backlash against his views and against the growing child protection movement. He may have furthered our understanding of the medical and moral complexities of infant mortality in general, and SIDS in particular, but angry pressure groups were formed by parents under suspicion and others who sympathized with them. (And don't we all sympathize with the outrage of those who claim to have been unjustly accused?)

The groups complained to the GMC about Professor Southall. The GMC took their protests to its Medical Practitioners' Tribunal Service. He was judged unfit to practise and struck off. It took him many years and a Court of Appeal decision to overturn this verdict. His condemnation by the GMC received wide coverage: his subsequent complete exoneration went almost unreported.

The Sally Clark case perhaps charts the history of our relationship with SIDS. Fashions in thinking should have no place in the world of scientific truth, but they certainly do. Ten years earlier she would have been regarded as simply a tragic figure for losing two babies. By the time her first son died, SIDS was declining but still a widely given cause of death. By the time her second son died, thinking had progressed further and any pathologist in the land would take into account the full circumstances of the case. The cause of death actually given was that the baby had been shaken, and this reflected the topicality of shaken baby syndrome at that time. Overall, the case revealed our deep new suspicion of mothers when their babies died suddenly. Her successful appeal may have reflected a public reconsideration of that level of suspicion.

In fact, although the pathologist involved certainly made errors of recording and disclosure, the medical evidence was extremely complex and controversial and huge numbers of experts lined up to disagree with each other in court on almost every aspect of both children's deaths. The truth in the Clark case, as in so many, proved to be not solid but a rather unpredictable liquid. The courts wanted honesty and truth and then chose to be selective and make their own assessments of highly complex medical issues.

No one emerged unscathed from the tragedy of the Clark case. For forensic pathologists, it was certainly a horrible reminder of the huge responsibilities of our profession.

# 32

Much as I loved life on the Isle of Man, after a couple of years I began to miss the cut and thrust of day-to-day forensic pathology. I missed the camaraderie in the mortuary and at crime scenes, the sense of a close-knit team working together. I recalled the great humanity of all involved, while the startling evidence of cruel, murderous inhumanity lay before us.

Committee work began to fill that gap. In particular, I was involved in producing guidelines to help the police and other authorities deal with a new challenge which was caused by the growing use of crack-cocaine. This drug can produce an extraordinary mental state in some users which makes them as strong as an ox and twice as dangerous. How to restrain these powerful, dangerous people to safeguard the public – without actually killing them? Helping to solve this problem was worthwhile, good work, but it was not like solving a problem at the mortuary. Now, I always seemed to be once removed from the body, from the scene of the crime, from the coalface.

Then, in 2004 I became engrossed in one of the most interesting and high-profile public inquiries underway at that time. It arose from events seven years earlier and many miles away.

*

I had not been the Home Office pathologist on call on the weekend of 31 August 1997: that fell to my colleague at St George's, Rob Chapman. In the early hours of that morning, the Princess of Wales and Dodi Al Fayed died in a road traffic accident in a Paris tunnel, he at the scene and she in hospital after an operation. The bodies were flown into RAF Northolt the same day and the then coroner for West London, John Burton, who by chance also happened to be the coroner for the Royal Household, assumed responsibility for them. That evening, surrounded by high-level police officers, evidence officers, a crime-scene manager, the coroner, Met police photographers and mortuary assistants, and with still more officers holding back the public outside, Rob carried out the post-mortems in Fulham. Both had died from injuries sustained in the accident.

The questions over those two deaths have never gone away. In a bid to stem the inevitable tide of conspiracy theories, a police inquiry was opened in 2004. It was led by Sir John Stevens, then commissioner of the Metropolitan Police, later Lord Stevens, and its aim was to establish whether or not there were grounds for treating the deaths as anything other than a road traffic accident. The new coroner to the Royal Household, Michael Burgess, suggested I act as forensic pathologist to this inquiry. Of course, both bodies had been long buried, and so it was my job to review the evidence my colleagues had produced in 1997.

There has famously been much speculation about the cause of the accident, but I don't think there is any doubt about the fact that Dodi and Diana left the back door of the Ritz in the hotel's Mercedes driven by Henri Paul and, crossing Paris at speed, pursued by photographers, their car hit the thirteenth concrete pillar in the Alma Tunnel at over 6omph.

If a car comes to a dead stop after such an impact, unless restrained by seat belts, the bodies of the people in the car don't stop with the vehicle. They continue forward and hit the windscreen, the dashboard or the people in front of them. Diana and Dodi, in the back seats, were not wearing seat belts. Nor was the driver. He hit the steering wheel and his injuries reflected that but, micro-seconds later, he was also hit from behind by Dodi, who was a big man and who was still travelling at over 6omph. Henri Paul effectively acted as Dodi's airbag and he died instantly. So did Dodi.

Diana was slightly more fortunate because the Al Fayeds' bodyguard, Trevor Rees-Jones, was sitting on the right of the driver, in front of her. Bodyguards don't usu-ally wear seat belts as they restrict movement, but evidently Rees-Jones, maybe because he was alarmed by Henri Paul's driving or maybe because he realized an impact was likely, put on his belt at the last minute. Belts are designed to give gradually while they restrain. So he was held by the belt and partially padded by the car's airbag, which by now had inflated, as Diana's body catapulted forward from the back seat. She was much lighter than Dodi and Rees-Jones's belt would have absorbed some of the extra force. This slightly lessened the energy of the impact for her and so, more protected than Dodi, she actually suf-fered just a few broken bones and a small chest injury.

Since Dodi Al Fayed and Henri Paul were clearly dead

when the ambulance arrived, the paramedics rightly turned to the injured. They did not recognize Diana, who is reported to have been talking. Trevor Rees-Jones had taken the double whammy of his own weight forcing him forward and Diana's weight hitting him from behind and he seemed much more seriously hurt. Of course, he was therefore taken out first. Diana was anyway effectively trapped behind the front passenger seat until he was removed.

Rees-Jones, as the more seriously injured party, was put in the first ambulance. Diana was then extracted from the car and taken to hospital as an emergency. No one knew that she had a tiny tear in a vein in one of her lungs. Anatomically, this site is hidden away, deep in the centre of the chest. Veins, of course, are not subject to the same high-pressure pumping as arteries. They bleed much more slowly, in fact they bleed so slowly that identifying the problem is hard enough and, if it is identified, repairing it is even harder.

To the ambulance services, she initially seemed injured but stable, particularly as she was able to communicate. While everyone focused on Rees-Jones, however, the vein was slowly bleeding into her chest. In the ambulance, she gradually lost consciousness. When she suffered a cardiac arrest, every effort was made to resuscitate her and in hospital she went into surgery, where they did identify the problem and attempted to repair the vein. But, sadly, by then it was too late. Her initial period of consciousness and initial survival after the accident is characteristic of a tear to a vital vein. Her specific injury is so rare that in my entire career I don't believe I've seen another. Diana's was a very small injury – but in the wrong place.

Her death is a classic example of the way we say, after almost every death: if only. *If only* she had hit the seat at a slightly different angle. *If only* she had been thrown forward 10mph more slowly. *If only* she had been put in an ambulance immediately. But the biggest *if only*, in Diana's case, was within her own control. *If only* she had been wearing a seat belt. Had she been restrained, she would probably have appeared in public two days later with a black eye, perhaps a bit breathless from the fractured ribs and with a broken arm in a sling.

The pathology of her death is, I believe, indisputable. But around that tiny, fatal tear in a pulmonary vein are woven many other facts, some of which are sufficiently opaque to allow a multitude of theories to blossom.

The conspiracy theorists, particularly Dodi's father, Mohammed Al Fayed, believe the crash was no accident but had been arranged. The most widely held proposition is that the couple were killed because Diana was about to embarrass the British establishment by announcing a pregnancy. Since I did not carry out her post-mortem myself, I cannot categorically say that she was not pregnant. Rob Chapman has been examined and cross-examined on this point and he has explained that there was no indication of pregnancy: bodily changes would have been detectable perhaps two but certainly three weeks after conception, even before she herself would have been aware of pregnancy.

Some people have asked me whether Rob could have been persuaded to lie. The answer is an emphatic 'no'. He would never dispense with the engrained methods of a lifetime and agree to obscure the truth from a post-mortem (and neither, for that matter, would I).

The conspiracy theories, however, did not rest entirely on Diana's alleged pregnancy. Any number of reasons have been proposed to explain why the car crashed that night and the theories have been fuelled by the various anomalies of the case.

First, there was the presence of a second car, a white Fiat Uno, which appears to have collided initially with the Ritz's Mercedes before the Mercedes hit the pillar. However, no one has ever discovered what happened because neither the car nor its driver – despite extensive searches throughout France and Europe – has ever been found.

Then there is the anomaly concerning the chauffeur, Henri Paul. His blood samples revealed him to be drunk, but this was hotly disputed by his family and by some of those who were with him shortly before the crash. There were accusations that someone else's blood had replaced Paul's, partly because his sample contained traces of a drug used to treat intestinal worms in children. Paul had neither worms nor children. However, the drug is also commonly used to 'cut' cocaine – although Paul had clearly taken no cocaine, at least not that night or even for a few days earlier. In addition, carbon monoxide levels were exceptionally, although not lethally, high in Paul's blood, and no one could satisfactorily explain that either.

Rather unusually, Diana's body had been embalmed. A French undertaker arrived at the hospital to do this and no one has ever really explained why he was called or by whom: certainly not by the pathologist at the hospital in

Paris. Probably the explanation is that embalming is a usual procedure for a member of the royal family, but since the bodies were flown immediately back to the UK and Rob carried out post-mortems within twenty-four hours of their deaths, there was no real need for the French to introduce preservation fluids into Diana's body. By doing so, they compromised all toxicology results. Some people saw this as suspicious action, but since neither Diana nor Dodi was driving it is very hard to see what significance any toxicology from them would have had.

After a lot of diplomatic wrangling and armed with many questions we, the police team and I, went to Paris. The French authorities did not greet us warmly, or even very helpfully but we saw the crash site and eventually even the car itself. Other specialists were trying to explain the carbon monoxide in Paul's blood and they immediately began to examine the airbag but my role, of course, took me to the mortuary.

Here I met Professor Dominique Lecomte, the charming pathologist who had the misfortune to be on duty that night. She had carried out the post-mortem on Henri Paul. She spoke good English until I started to discuss the post-mortem and whether possible lapses in recording systems meant the blood samples could have belonged to anyone other than Henri Paul. At that point, she said little more and insisted on speaking only through an interpreter, and often looked for advice to the lawyer who sat next to her.

I hope she understood how much I sympathized and empathized with her. A routine Saturday night in a big-city mortuary includes the odd road traffic accident, unlucky drunks, the victims of crime and brawls. In Paris, pathologists do not routinely deal with these over the weekend; they start performing their post-mortems on Monday morning. Professor Lecomte was therefore asleep at home in the middle of the night when she was dragged off into a situation of sudden and immense pressure. The world's most photographed face had died in a car crash and her driver and boyfriend had also arrived at the mortuary. Outside, governments, family and the international press were howling for the professor's conclusions.

The general rule when presented with a high-profile death is to stop. Do everything slowly. Carry out all procedures correctly and in strict sequence. It is worth following these rules because a celebrity death means that your every action will be questioned for a long time afterwards in public and in private. During the event itself, you are under pressure to get things done right now. In half the usual time and with half the usual information. To give simple answers immediately to complex medical questions. I have learned the hard way that no one says thank you in these cases. Ever. The only comments that are made are critical – you either did something you shouldn't have done or (more commonly) you failed to do something that, in retrospect, you possibly should have done.

Unfortunately, pathologists in this situation sometimes do bow to the immense pressure placed on them to hurry, to cut corners, to accept 'the obvious'. They do things out of sequence and may behave in an uncharacteristically haphazard way. I am not suggesting that Professor Lecomte carried out her post-mortem haphazardly. I think she did a good job, and, although I was later to uncover some errors, I have no criticism of her. And I can very well understand her defensiveness when a British pathologist arrived to ask insistent questions about how well she followed her own procedures after she was woken suddenly for a particularly demanding night's work seven years earlier.

The Stevens inquiry cost £4 million and resulted in a 900-page report, which was finally submitted at the end of 2006. It said, 'Our conclusion is that, on all the evidence available at this time, there was no conspiracy to murder any of the occupants of the car. This was a tragic accident.'

The report did nothing to stop the conspiracy theorists, certainly not Mohammed Al Fayed. In 2007, after much pressure, a full inquest was announced. I was called as an expert witness and this time the French were finally persuaded to produce more of their files. I had already seen Henri Paul's full post-mortem report, of course. Then, in late September, very close to the start of the inquest, the French authorities finally released the post-mortem photos of Henri Paul.

In 1997 police photographers used film cameras. The numbers on the negatives were reproduced on the back of the prints and this meant it was possible easily to follow the sequence of the pictures that were taken in the mortuary. The first of the photographs clearly showed that Paul had been placed face down at the start of the examination. In pathology you are taught to look at the whole of the microscope slide – there's always the chance of a tiny bit of cancer at one edge. The same rule applies to photographs. Ignore the blindingly obvious to begin with and look at the background. So I looked at the background of the Paul photographs and they showed a row of empty glass bottles, lined up and waiting for his blood samples, on the sink beside the mortuary table behind the body.

Professor Lecomte's report described a huge area of bleeding in the back of Paul's neck – probably caused by the impact from Dodi's body. Nothing unusual about that. But it was very odd that I could see more of the blood bottles filling with each sequential picture. There were a number that were evidently full before the body was turned over ready for the chest and abdomen to be opened.

That would have no great significance except that, in her report, Professor Lecomte states that the blood samples she submitted were taken from the heart. And not from the neck.

Of course, she might first have taken samples from the neck as a precaution and then discarded them when she turned the body over and found she was able to take cardiac samples instead (cardiac samples are regarded as acceptable: in fact, femoral samples are the best). That would be good practice. But only if she recorded her actions.

Or she may have labelled blood samples from the neck as being from the heart. It doesn't matter so much where the samples are taken from. Saying where they are taken from does matter. The site of sampling can significantly affect the toxicologists' interpretation of the results, and incorrect labelling can lead to great inaccuracies.

You might take this as an oversight. You might take it as an indication of poor record-keeping. But, in a case like this where every tiny event matters, it can give rise to many more questions about sampling sites, labelling of bottles and security of transfer – and it certainly fuelled the accusations that these weren't Paul's blood samples anyway. Residual blood in the samples was tested and proved to be Henri Paul's but that did not end the matter because there were missing samples, spilt samples, samples that had been shared with other labs ... leaving enough room for doubt for those who really wanted to raise questions.

It was for the jury to decide the significance, if any, of the evidence I gave to the inquest. This was a large-scale affair, presided over by Lord Justice Scott Baker, who had been appointed coroner specifically to this inquest. He was represented by three barristers, Mohammed Al Fayed by three, there were two for the Ritz hotel in Paris and two for the family of Henri Paul. In addition, the Metropolitan Police was represented by three barristers and the Intelligence Service and Foreign Office by two. Other interested parties, including Diana's sons and her sister, also had lawyers at the inquest.

Although, of course, there was considerable media attention at certain points, most days the lawyers heavily outnumbered the totality of both press and public.

Questioning of the witnesses, as usual at an inquest, came first from the coroner's barrister – but there was often cross-examination from one or more of the others. Every tiny detail of that night and the months leading up to it was examined. My own contribution was minimal but, I think, important to the outcome. I was asked what my overall impression of the events was. My conclusion? A simple, high-speed, alcohol-related, road traffic accident.

The jury's final verdict astonished no one and satisfied many:

> Unlawful killing, grossly negligent driving of the following vehicles and of the Mercedes. The crash was caused or contributed to by the speed and manner of driving of the Mercedes, the speed and manner of driving of the following vehicles, the impairment of the judgement of the driver of the Mercedes through alcohol.

I wish that Professor Lecomte had not been so resistant to Shepherd's charm offensive and had talked a little more: her silence does mean that, pathologically speaking, there is a slight lack of clarity. But that doesn't mean I can credit conspiracy theories. I do not believe that what happened in the mortuary that mad night was part of a wider plan to murder a woman in such a haphazard way and then hide the evidence. Simply, Professor Lecomte made small errors under pressure, which, in a case without so many seeking fodder for their theories, would not have been significant. I entirely concur with the jury's verdict.

## 33

In 2006 Tony Blair was still prime minister, there was a summer heatwave and *CSI* was named the world's most popular TV programme. Chris was almost a vet and Anna halfway through medical school. On the Isle of Man, *Simpson's Forensic Medicine, Twelfth Edition* had been not just finished but published. My pride in it was tempered by the sense of finality the book's completion gave me. Reading the third edition had started my career. Was the writing of the twelfth edition a sign my career was ending?

I still had plenty of work: sitting on committees, giving opinions on complex cases and evidence at public inquiries. But life was very different from that busy world I'd known before, a world that always had at its centre a body, demise unexplained, name perhaps unknown.

Occasionally I began to experience a sense of ennui as I walked the hills with the dogs and stared at the sea. What was it? It took a while for me to recognize something I have barely experienced in the whole of my life. Boredom. Or was it loneliness? I hardly knew what that was, either.

Alone together after some buzzing social event, Jen and I didn't seem to have much to say to each other. There was no need to discuss the children like we used to now they were grown, and the cottage renovations were finished so there was nothing much to say about that either. Jen bought some sheep and started to learn how to manage her flock. I tried to develop an interest in sheep, too. But the fact was, much as I loved our home overlooking the sea, it had begun to seem very silent. I even welcomed the noisy storms that banged on the windows and battered the roof, because they made the house feel so alive.

When we moved to the island we had both thought there would be some part-time work there, perhaps for me in the mortuary and surely for Jen in a dermatology clinic. But this proved closed to us due to island medical politics and Jen ended up spending one week a month working at a clinic on the mainland. In 2006 I was offered forensic work as a weekend locum in Liverpool. And I took it.

Maybe I had limped away from London to the Isle of Man feeling battered by my working life. By its politics, its administrative responsibilities, the interpersonal complexities of the new world of private pathology. Only now did I realize what I missed: the very heart of my work, that is, the dead and their mysteries. Standing in the Liverpool mortuary in my scrubs, with my PM40 sharp in my hand, I even felt renewed professional excitement for my first patient, one smelly and drunken knife victim who had been found in a rubbish chute. This was standby forensic work for the police and I stayed in a hotel for one weekend a month in order to do it. Sometimes I was called out to a stream of homicides and sometimes, to my great disappointment, nothing happened at all.

I hadn't been away from hands-on work for long, just

about two years, but we seemed to be in a new era of forensic pathology. The changes weren't dramatic so much as a continuation of developments I had first begun to notice in London.

Bodies were and are changing. Body fat has increased exponentially in the population, so that unless a patient is homeless or has died of cancer or is so old or poor they could not eat, few are the same shape as the dead of the 1980s when I started practising. Looking back at forensic photos from that era I am astonished at how thinness was then the norm.

Bodies also look different because they are so much more ornate: once tattoos were for fighting men and sailors. Now it seems that the majority of mortuary admissions have piercings or tattoos. In addition, self-harm was almost unknown then and now I am amazed at the number of bodies, particularly the young, which arrive in the mortuary with old, self-inflicted cuts and lacerations: it tells me about their life and about changing society but nothing about their death, the causes of which are generally not directly related to self-harm.

For the pathologist in the 1980s, HIV and hepatitis were becoming the acknowledged enemy, and they still are. But by the time I returned to work from the Isle of Man, TB was an occupational hazard for anyone working in a mortuary and I knew several pathologists and mortuary staff who had caught it. TB is much more prevalent than you would guess and, not uncommonly, even at post-mortem, we have no idea that we are about to be exposed to a highly infectious disease which every other doctor has mistaken for a simple pneumonia.

Post-mortem reports have changed too. When I started, three pages was considered adequate. When I returned, I was criticized for producing anything less than ten, and they were expected to be discursive, explaining the workings of the human body at length.

Back in the 1990s, DNA started to make a significant contribution to forensic work, and forensic science soon overtook forensic pathology as the field's major contribution to crime-cracking. Before I left, the police had begun to ask us to wear gloves at the scene of a crime. By the time I came back, it was gloves, boots, white Tylex suit (hood up), and a face mask too. DNA analysis had become so much more sensitive that now we knew just breathing, just talking, sprays saliva with DNA everywhere. Gone are the days of the pathologist and senior investigating officer walking around the scene in their office clothes discussing the case. The white suits are certainly not designed for ease of dressing, nor for comfort, and it's always embarrassing to try to put one on when the world's press is filming you. But it is so good to take them off at the end of the scene examination and put them in an evidence bag – yes, even the suits are kept for trace evidence now.

In court I had for years noticed how cases for the prosecution were becoming less meticulously researched and organized. Now, case conferences with counsel are a thing of the past. There is never a phone call: not from the police, the Crown Prosecution Service or even counsel. If I am lucky, I'll get ten minutes with the QC before I go into the witness box. More often, barristers don't have a clue what answers I'm going to give when they stand up and start to question me. Often, they don't even allow me the chance to tell the jury who I am and why the years have particularly qualified me to discuss this subject: 'Dr Shepherd, you're a registered medical practitioner, tell me what you found on your examination of the body.'

The days of the thundering, bombastic QC were already ending when I left London: that defence QC who gave me such a hard time over the rent boy's all-over bruising was already a relic from the past and now such barristers are almost completely gone. Presumably for economic reasons, the Crown Prosecution Service seems to use junior barristers rather than much more expensive QCs. Of course, experienced, although not so overtly thundering, QCs are still out there, and they are nearly always working for the defence.

Courts are much more interested in expert witnesses giving what is now called 'evidence-based' testimony rather than experience-based, no matter how much experience we have. Judges have occasionally stopped me answering important questions fully with a curt, 'Just give us a yes or no, Dr Shepherd.' Often when I am responding to a long and detailed question from counsel.

The essentially self-employed structure of forensic pathology in England and Wales that was introduced as I left London has removed almost completely the possibility of forensic research. Most of us do not now work or teach at universities: forensic medicine no longer even has a place on the medical-school curriculum. Research has anyway been effectively neutered by the Human Tissue Authority's insistence that families of the deceased give consent before samples, even minute samples, can be used for research purposes. How then, you may ask, can the answers we give to the courts be 'evidence-based'?

There will always be homicides and suicides and accidents, but now the routine forensic caseload will, increasingly, include negligence and 'safeguarding' issues in nursing homes. It will certainly include a large number of deaths from drug overdose. And, shamefully, there are many more deaths in custody, which speaks volumes about our jails: 316 in the year to March 2017, of which ninety-seven were suicides. In the same year, there were in jails over 40,000 incidents of self-harm and over 26,000 assaults. And these figures are rising alarmingly year on year.

The most shocking change I noticed on my return is that forensic pathologists are called to investigate a death less often. The cost and administration of opening an inquest seems to encourage some coroners to overlook an element of doubt. If there 'might be' a natural cause and a doctor 'might be' willing to sign a form, many coroners will accept that without too much inquiry. Sadly, the need for the police to pay a standard fee, admittedly several thousand pounds, to a forensic pathologist, may be enough to persuade them that a death (especially, it sometimes seems, one close to the end of the financial year) really is not so suspicious after all and can be dealt with by a local, non-forensic pathologist instead of one of the forty or so specialists registered by the Home Office.

Most people would agree that a civilized society should endeavour always to find, no matter what it costs, the true cause of death. The cost of the trials, the inquest and public inquiry into the death of Stephen Lawrence should serve to remind anyone in any doubt that it is far, far better and far, far cheaper to do all things properly at the start.

I found that I enjoyed being back at the coalface in Liverpool, different though it looked. I was sometimes invited to lecture on the mainland by medical bodies or other professional groups, and I enjoyed that too. At the end of these lectures, interested people usually came forward to ask me questions. After one lecture in London, a forensic paediatrician chatted to me about my work. A forensic paediatrician can expect to see cases of child abuse, both physical and sexual, and this was, in fact, the paediatrician's specialization: not death, but the protection of the living. She asked me questions about bruising and we agreed that, with our combined knowledge, we really should write an academic paper on the subject. Our work overlapped in that problem area between my research into whether a child had died naturally and her research into whether living siblings were in danger, and we met several times to discuss the paper on bruising during my subsequent trips to the mainland.

On the Isle of Man, our house became more and more silent. Jen shepherded her flock. I studied my papers.

One day, she said, 'We really ought to discuss our marriage.'

And I said, 'What marriage? It hardly seems to exist.'

That was how it ended. One night in February. Not with a bang but a whimper. With little talk. But much pain. After thirty years.

How quickly, in comparison to its length, the marriage

unravelled. Perhaps every entity has a limited lifetime. Perhaps senescence is built into relationships just as it is built into the human body. It seemed to me there was simply nothing left of this marriage of ours but it was impossible to say this, to think it, without inflicting pain and engendering fury. There was the past and there were two children and a shared property and that, of course, all had to be discussed, often acrimoniously, always with much pain on both sides. But we shared so little else that I was sure, when the shouting was over and the hurt receding, that better lives lay ahead for both of us.

Jen issued papers to divorce me and the process was complete within one year.

It was not obvious to me at this time that I would fall in love with the forensic paediatrician I had been meeting to discuss our work on bruising, let alone that she would become my future wife, but I was never able to persuade Jen of my innocence in this. It was true I was spending time with someone whom I knew to be of special warmth, empathy and intelligence, but there had been no further planning on my part. Nor on Linda's. She had been widowed when her three daughters were very small and for some years now she had been in a relationship. That relationship and my marriage both ended with mess and fury.

Despite her determination to divorce me, Jen suffered greatly. Our separation caused considerable unhappiness to our children, too, who also, I think, wrongly suspected that I had simply found Linda and dumped Jen. Anna, almost a doctor herself now, during the period when her mother's pain was greatest and her anger red hot, declared that one thing she would never become is a pathologist like her father.

I am glad to say that Jen did find happiness with a new partner. And in September 2008 Linda and I were married. This added another family to mine and I found myself back in the world of teenagers as well as busy, elderly parents. No matter how loving and welcoming a new family, relationships between each individual, between the two families, must be built slowly, over years. We have applied ourselves to this and the result, I hope, is a strong and loving extended unit.

Since that time, I have lived and worked as a forensic pathologist in the north of England. Life here is rich and varied: stimulating work, a warm and loving home, interesting holidays, surprise expeditions, a shared aeroplane to fly, five children between us and, for me, two grandchildren now.

My son, Chris, is a vet, specializing in horses. He now lives abroad, where the landscapes and perhaps the mindscapes are wider. Anyway, he has certainly escaped poor pay and dark mornings. And he is following me in one way: by learning to fly.

Anna is a consultant histopathologist and, yes, she does have a keen interest in post-mortem and forensic medicine and even works for some of the coroners I worked for years ago. We chat often about cases: I seek her advice on 'newfangled' tests and she seeks my opinion on causes of death. She changed her name when she married and no one can say that her father's name is connected in any way with her achievements. But probably no one would, because she is obviously very much her own person. Anna doesn't find herself torn between modern practice and a desire to be Keith Simpson. No, Anna's world is much more complex and accountable than the one I knew at her age. I see that world as less colourful. But she doesn't. She never knew Simpson's limitless horizons.

I would say that my knowledge of death has helped me appreciate the importance of life's small pleasures and I bask in them: a loved child running excitedly through a carpet of red and yellow fallen leaves, or tracing a finger with deep fascination along the wrinkles on my face, a fire ablaze while rain throws itself against the window, a dog hurtling towards me to welcome me home, a gentle hand placed lovingly on mine. I am no stranger to joy. I know that joy can be truly experienced only by those who have known adversity. And adversity is an inevitability.

# 34

One morning the phone rang and an angry voice cried, 'Have you read this crap? Have you?'

The voice was instantly recognizable as Ellie's. She is a paediatric pathologist with whom I'd worked on the occasional case. And the crap she was referring to? We'd together performed a post-mortem on a baby named Noah eighteen months ago and given SIDS as the cause of death. I'd noticed there was something new about this case in my inbox, waiting to be opened.

Ellie was unstoppable.

'How can we have missed lip injuries and fractures on the posterior ribs too? How? The lips were resuscitation injuries or I'm Naomi Campbell! And we looked and didn't see any posterior rib fractures and neither did the radiologist. How is it that this person can just look at the photographs and find suffocation injuries and old fractures? Tell me that, Dick!'

The parents of the late Baby Noah now had another baby. Social services evidently felt there was enough doubt hanging over the earlier SIDS death to safeguard the new baby by removing her from the parents' care. Their application to do so was heading for the Family Court. Recently the court had asked for copies of our report on Baby Noah, our notes and the post-mortem photographs. And evidently, all this had now been reviewed by another pathologist who specialized in working for that court. I clicked on the email. Yes, here were his comments.

'Ellie, he's surely not saying that we missed . . .'

'He *is*!'

'I'll look at the pictures and call you back.'

I felt sick. Was it possible that I had examined a dead baby who had been abused and murdered and failed to spot the evidence for this? And actually given SIDS, exonerating the parents and endangering any future babies they might have? And had the evidence been so obvious that eighteen months later another pathologist could pick it up just from the photographs?

I dug out the file. Baby Noah was many cases ago. I tried to remember that day.

I had been called to the mortuary by the police because the mother had found her baby dead in the morning. Waiting for me in the lounge area next to the inevitable mortuary fish tank was Ellie – the post-mortem of a child whose death is suspicious must be carried out by two pathologists, one forensic, one paediatric. Ellie is good to work with: witty and wise, she demonstrates a 100 per cent certainty about her own conclusions that I secretly envy.

Now I flicked through my notes. The mother gave Baby Noah a bottle at 8 p.m. and, since he was sniffling, also some paracetamol. He went to sleep but had woken twice in the night. The first time, at about 2 a.m., the father had rocked him back to sleep. The second time was at 5 a.m. and the father was waking up anyway, since he was on an early shift. He settled the baby and left the house at 6 a.m. without really waking the mother. At 7 a.m. she had found the baby dead. She ran, screaming, into the street. A neighbour, who had seen resuscitation techniques demonstrated on *EastEnders*, ran in and attempted to revive the baby until the ambulance crew arrived to take over. Without success.

Pictures of the home had shown the disorder one expects to find where there is a new baby. There was little furniture because the place was dominated by large, plastic toys of the kind Grandma buys at Argos. The fridge was nearly empty except for milk and leftover takeaway cartons. Upstairs the bedroom was almost filled by the bed and cot: there were piles of baby clothes on the remaining floor area.

Most notable for us as pathologists was the temperature of the place. We saw pictures of the boiler thermostat downstairs set to thirty degrees and pictures of the bedroom radiators on max. The police had commented on how hot the house was. There is, of course, a strong association between SIDS and overheated babies.

Some time after we had completed our post-mortem report, a number of anomalies and untruths emerged. Muslim neighbours were shocked to find their bins full of empty alcohol bottles and mentioned this to the police. Noah's parents later admitted that they had disposed of these bottles in the night. Toxicology extrapolated the father's blood alcohol level at the time the baby was supposed to have first woken at 200mg/100ml, two and a half times the drink-drive limit. And the same tests revealed that both parents had been smoking cannabis.

The father had an old GBH conviction after a fight, but there was no history of domestic violence. The baby had an old shoulder injury, but this could easily have been caused by his very difficult birth. The police were clearly suspicious of this couple but could not really articulate why – although they did find out that the house was so hot because there was a small cannabis farm in the loft. The ambulance crew strongly suggested that the baby had been dead for a few hours, not just one as the mother insisted. But they weren't sure. And all the marks on Baby Noah's body could be explained by the untrained resuscitation techniques of the neighbour and the subsequent prolonged attempts of the ambulance crew.

Ellie and I had to agree on a cause of death. As the paediatric pathologist, she was going to write the report and I would make any corrections and then sign it.

Ellie was sure she knew what she wanted to say.

'SIDS, Dick. It's SIDS.'

'But there's too much about it that's not quite right. I'd rather give "Unascertained".'

'We're not here to pass judgement on them for having a few cannabis plants in the attic, for heaven's sake. Or for liking a drink. They're obviously not a chaotic pair of addicts. The father has a regular job, the baby was healthy and well cared for, they turned up for all their health-visitor appointments and vaccinations, there was a supportive wider family – the grandma, the sister. No, don't let's leave "Unascertained" hanging over a young couple who're simply poor and doing their best.'

SIDS it was, then.

Except now another pathologist had looked at the post-mortem pictures and decided it wasn't.

I put the pictures up on the screen. Here were the baby's lips. They were redder than I remembered and the marks on them were more prominent, but there was no swelling or bruising. These were injuries caused during resuscitation. I then looked for the serial pictures of the inside of the chest showing the baby's ribs. Sure enough, I could see some whitening in some areas. Which might indicate old fractures. Or was it just the glare from the photographer's flash?

I phoned Ellie back: 'The lips look redder and more marked in these pictures than they really were and there are actually some areas that look white on the back of the ribs –' I could hear her exploding so I went on quickly. 'We know that's not how it was. If you look at the pictures closely enough, you'll see some of the other organs are odd colours and there seem to be flash reflections littering the images. It's the photos.'

'Who took them?' she roared. 'Who took these rubbish pictures?'

I remembered how a SOCO had stepped forward rather shyly with the camera. Had it been his first 'proper' job? He had asked his senior for advice several times and then the auxiliary flash had stopped working, and he eventually had to rely on the camera's own built-in flash.

When I looked through the rest of the photos I saw their quality was so poor that Baby Noah's white nappy had a distinct blue hue. Why hadn't I noticed this earlier?

'Don't worry, Ellie,' I said. 'It must just be a technical problem with the flash and it's been made worse by the low resolution they've used to store the images.'

'I'm not worried,' she told me coolly. 'Nope. I'm very, very angry. This pathologist who's criticized us doesn't do post-mortems himself. And he certainly wasn't present at this one. The other forensic pathologists who looked at the body on behalf of the family agreed with us, didn't they? How dare he challenge us when –?'

'Because . . . well, have you read the rest of the file yet?'

'No I have not!'

'Because they've now found out all sorts of things about the parents. Stuff they didn't know before. Which gives a different picture. We thought they were young and struggling and trying to make ends meet with their little cannabis farm in the loft . . . but now it turns out that the father already had a baby with someone else, down south somewhere. About four years ago. And it died. SIDS was given as the cause of death.'

That silenced even Ellie for a moment.

I said, 'It doesn't help that he's a former heroin addict who until quite recently had a methadone script. I wish they'd told us all that.'

'Oh, go on. Just victimize a man when he's doing his best to get clean. Was he on methadone when the baby died?'

'No.'

'There you are, then.'

'When he met the mother and had the baby he was really trying to live a better life; that's how I read his police interviews.'

'Exactly, and if we took every baby away from every recovering heroin addict, there wouldn't be any children left in some parts of town.'

'Listen, Ellie, we'll go to court, give our evidence, explain that the photos are faulty and we're sure the child did not have old fractures, explain that the radiologist agrees with us, and that will be an end to it.'

'It won't be so simple. We've given SIDS and they don't want to hear that. I think they just want to take the next child away. It's quite clear they believe Baby Noah was killed.'

'Courts are briefed to find the truth, not what they want to hear.'

There was a loud noise halfway between a laugh and a snort and then she was gone.

The court case really didn't worry me. In fact, I was quite curious. The Family Courts have retained their mystery for me as for everyone else because until now only my written evidence had been used. These courts deal with such personal, sensitive issues that they are absolutely closed to press and public: no one without a direct reason to be there is admitted, not even close relatives of the deceased or their family.

Ellie was waiting for me outside. She looked nervous.

'You should see how many people are in there.'

'How? Virtually no one's allowed in apart from lawyers and witnesses.'

'There are a trillion lawyers. The mother has a solicitor, a junior barrister and a QC. So does the father. So does the local authority. So does the new baby! Not three months old and she already has three lawyers! So that's twelve of them for starters, then there are loads of officials. Dick, now they're cutting back legal aid for criminal cases, lawyers must be into the Family Courts like vultures. Cases last for weeks here!'

I thought she was probably exaggerating.

'Just as well there's only one judge, then,' I said. 'Sounds as though there wouldn't be room for a jury too.'

But once inside the courtroom I saw that the place was indeed thronged with lawyers. No one was technically on trial, of course. The defendant's box was empty. It was one judge's job to decide whether a baby should be taken into care or perhaps safeguarded in some other way. There were lots of factors he would take into account but whether, on the balance of probabilities, a parent had injured or killed Baby Noah was the central question. No trial then, just an investigation into the truth. But with a full adversarial presentation, barristers each questioning, cross-examining and arguing their clients' case. I recalled that, as Aeschylus allegedly said, the first casualty of war is truth.

I was allowed to sit in the courtroom during Ellie's testimony and so was able to see both parents. They sat separately and did not look at each other. They had a new baby but they seemed not to be together: of course, their legal teams would each now be playing the blame game.

The mother was angry. Overweight, barely moving, her face large as though swollen, she managed to create a sense of noise around her, swearing into the ear of her solicitor and sometimes out loud into the quiet courtroom. The father was very thin and he sniffed and fidgeted constantly as though the proceedings were keeping him from something more important. Like a fix. If they had really killed Baby Noah they were not to be pitied. But if they hadn't . . . they looked like two unhappy, unloved people who perhaps had struggled to learn to love their baby.

In the witness box, Ellie was losing her cool. I watched

with growing concern as barrister after barrister attempted to question her competence in giving SIDS as Baby Noah's cause of death. When they had finished mauling her, I knew what was coming next.

Almost as soon as I had taken the oath, the first barrister began by pointing out that the baby had in fact been wearing a blue Babygro with green rabbits on it – annoyingly, Ellie had reversed the colours in the post-mortem report and I had failed to notice that the rabbits weren't blue when I checked it. She had also made one small mistake over a date, reversing the month and day, which I had, once again, failed to notice. Not major errors but it was the usual quibbling at the start of an examination designed to challenge my competence and undermine my confidence before the big fight. And the big fight was, of course, going to be the baby's lip injuries and the alleged fractures to the posterior ribs.

'Dr Shepherd, do you agree that old, now healed, fractures to the baby's back ribs would be a strong indicator of abuse over his short lifetime?'

'I agree that, if there had been healed fractures, abuse would be one possible explanation.'

'Did you look for such fractures?'

'All the ribs were examined extremely carefully . . .'

I pointed out that the photos were poor and did not represent what we actually saw. This was brushed aside: 'We can all see that the back ribs were previously fractured in the photos, Dr Shepherd. So why can't you?'

We had the same conversation about the lip injuries.

'Just look at the photographs, Dr Shepherd! The presence of injuries is obvious!'

I explained that, because of the way the images were stored, transmitted and then printed on a poor quality printer, they could not be relied upon. It was clear, though, that I wasn't making any progress. They could see what they could see. I was either blind or stupid not to accept that and – if I was either – I was obviously deliberately obfuscating to avoid the fact that I – we, Ellie and I – with seventy years of pathological experience between us, had dismissed suffocation injuries as resuscitation injuries.

There followed as demanding an afternoon as I have ever spent in the witness box of any court, including the Old Bailey. And, in a way, it was worse – instead of one hostile barrister, there were many, representing all sides, each attacking me from a different angle. I managed to hold my ground, acknowledging the possibility that we could have been wrong but saying it was highly unlikely that two experienced pathologists would have missed such clear evidence of abuse.

'Are you an osteopathologist, Dr Shepherd?'

'No, I am not.'

'But you were concerned about the baby's ribs, the evident fractures at the front?'

'Concerned that the fractures were open to interpretation, yes, but aware that violent resuscitation by an untrained neighbour had –'

'You were concerned, but not concerned enough to submit the ribs to an osteopathologist for his specialist comments?'

'It did not seem to me that he could shed any further light on the ribs. We had seen which ones were broken and we knew that –'

'You thought you knew as much as the specialist, is that it?'

'The radiologist said, in her opinion, there were no fractures at the back of the ribs. We had easily seen the fractures at the front. I felt the further knowledge of an osteopathologist would add nothing.'

'Wasn't that rather arrogant of you, Dr Shepherd?'

'I do not consider myself an arrogant person. I am sorry if I appear that way.'

Alexander Pope's lines appeared in my head as if my father had just inserted them there.

> But you, with Pleasure own your Errors past,
> And make each Day a Critick on the last.

'Do you admit the possibility that you were wrong to give SIDS?'

'Assessment of a cause of death in these cases is always very difficult, there's a very fine line. On the evidence we had when we wrote our reports, SIDS took precedence. Had we been given fuller information about the circumstances of the baby's life and death, I believe we would probably have chosen "Unascertained" instead.'

The surprise of my afternoon at the Family Court was not just the attacks on me professionally, but personally. The second surprise was the written judgment. It arrived some weeks later. I learned from it that there had been a series of witnesses in court over the weeks of the case who gave examples of how neglected Baby Noah had been by his parents. The mother had now emerged as an alcoholic, the father as a frequent drug abuser. The mother's sister and an aunt had been stepping in to help with Baby Noah, inadvertently promoting a false impression of the mother's competence to the health visitor and others. According to the judge, it was they who had ensured the baby was looked after and taken to his appointments and vaccinations.

He said that Baby Noah had been neglected and he was shocked by the refusal or inability of the two pathologists who examined the body to accept that they had missed such obvious and glaring marks of abuse – which could be seen in the photos by anyone. Indeed, he said the pathologists still seemed to think that SIDS might well be the cause of death. The judge did not make any mention that the photos were of, at best, variable quality. Nor of the lack of information provided to us about the parents on the day their baby died when we had carried out the post-mortem. Nor of any failure to update us as further information about the family was uncovered.

He went on to say that, on the balance of probabilities – which was the test he had to apply – he concluded that the father had killed Baby Noah. Under cross-examination it had been revealed that, on the night of the baby's death, large quantities of drink and some drugs had been consumed and when the baby cried, the father had responded. The judge supposed that he probably did this by pressing down on the baby's chest, and possibly his face, asphyxiating him and perhaps breaking his ribs. There was evidence, he said, from the baby's posterior ribs, that something like this had in fact happened before. On this occasion, the mother had asked him to do anything to stop the baby crying and, although she was aware that he was behaving harshly to Baby Noah, she did nothing to intervene. Therefore, no other child should be left in the care of either parent. Their new baby was to be taken from them for adoption.

I cannot imagine how the parents of Baby Noah felt on receiving that judgment. I was so crushed by it that I believe I actually gasped for breath. It was impossible that harsh words from a judge about a Home Office pathologist would not cause considerable repercussions. I had reached the age of sixty and had tried hard to work through medicine in the interests of justice all my life. And now it seemed that balance and justice were being withheld from me.

That night, I could not sleep. I could barely breathe. Such critical comments must require investigation and, as a Home Office pathologist, I must report them to the Home Office. Would the Home Office then investigate me? Refer me to the General Medical Council? The GMC can take away from doctors the right to practise if they are found guilty of serious misconduct.

The unfairness of this possibility made me sit up in bed. I was being accused of poor judgement on the basis of poor photos. Injuries on the lips and healed cracks in the posterior ribs could be evidence of old abuse but there had been no injuries to the lips and the fronts of the ribs that couldn't be explained by resuscitation, and no cracks at the backs of the ribs at all. I was sure of it, Ellie was sure of it, the radiologist was sure of it. We had said in our report that, although the injuries to the front ribs were probably caused by resuscitation, we could not exclude the possibility that they had been caused deliberately.

But then, of course, we had given SIDS as the cause of death.

Surely, surely, it was impossible that I would be struck off for such a thing?

When at last I slept, my dreams were a strange jumble of courtrooms and babies. The next day my night thoughts still shrouded me. Without thinking about the court case directly it nevertheless informed my every action. In my stomach, the patina of dread. In my head, a sense of crisis. Sitting at my desk that afternoon, tortured by inexplicable anxiety, I stopped fighting. I knew what was going to happen. It had started to happen flying over Hungerford recently. Then again after the Paris bombings. I had learned to clench my fist and with a supreme force of will almost keep myself away from the abyss. But now it opened right in front of me.

I shut my eyes. It was waiting for me. The bodies, piled high, the stench of decay and heat, young people who had been dancing when the bomb went off, when the boat went down, young people without hands, children exhumed in their coffins, babies' tiny bodies bearing helpless testament to man's inhumanity, charred bodies, drowned bodies, bodies severed on the railway track. A deep, deep pit of human suffering.

I looked up again. I blinked. I looked around my office. Computer, desk, pictures, files, dogs. All normal. It had been another of those quick trips to hell again, as sudden and shocking as an epileptic fit.

And anyway, I was back in the present now. I was going to get on with my work. Which was to write to the Home Office reporting the judge's comments about me in the Baby Noah case.

A short while later, the Home Office replied. They were already aware of the case and said they had been for some time. Although they hadn't bothered to let me know. The police officer involved in the case had reported me to them and they had decided to pass the file to the General Medical Council. I might, they said, wish to discuss the matter with my lawyer.

I most certainly did. She was reassuring but I was not reassured. At night my dreams were hideous. In the day, awake in my office, I fought with nightmares.

At last, a letter arrived. I opened it with shaking hands. I wanted it to tell me that the whole thing had been dismissed and that it was over.

It said I was under investigation by the General Medical Council. My competence had been called into question because of the cause of death given in Baby Noah's postmortem report, signed by me.

Then, all joy stopped. And those events that I had not been calling panic attacks? Well, even I had to admit that's exactly what they were.

I have spent my entire working life reviewing cases. Now *I* was a case. Now *I* was under review. The GMC is essentially a private court that investigates at its own pace and behind closed doors. It gives no information about the length of time it will take to resolve issues and does not communicate on the matter other than to issue edicts – to which I had to respond within a very short time frame.

I knew the GMC was quietly contacting colleagues, coroners, police officers, anyone who had worked with me, for their opinions of me and of my skills. The GMC did not say whether or when it might refer my case to the next level, the tribunal. I would be informed when that referral was made.

The tribunal is the Medical Practitioners Tribunal Service, which is independent of the GMC and adjudicates cases sent to it by the GMC. It hears evidence on oath, with examination and cross-examination by barristers, and they return a verdict on whether a doctor is fit to practise. Or not. It is, effectively, a court.

All this because another pathologist who worked for the Family Court suggested I made mistakes, that I missed obvious injuries and gave a cause of death for Baby Noah that he considered incorrect. Pathology is a combination of facts, experience and judgement. But the tribunal could ignore this and conclude from the accusations made that I was not trustworthy to determine how a child had died and therefore whether siblings were at risk. They could decide I should be 'struck off'. That is, removed from the register of doctors considered fit to practise.

Once the GMC investigation began, I started to experience, with renewed and alarming frequency, more panic attacks. Sequences of heart-stopping, heartbreaking images completely took over my mind.

I tried to adopt a detached, medical view of this. So, these ambushes had started when I was flying over Hungerford one day. Why exactly had they started, why exactly had they stopped? Obviously the GMC investigation had triggered their ugly and forceful return. Had this public doubting of a man who is supposed never to be wrong opened up a chasm of hidden fears? And were these fears now out of control?

There were no answers. Only images that inhabited my head suddenly and totally at the most unexpected moments. All I had to do was put some ice in Linda's drink and I was back in Bali, staring at the young bodies rotting beneath their bags of melting ice. There was no question of my opening any of the files piled in my office. Because inside them lurked pictures. And there were already too many pictures inside my head to manage. A sense of dread immobilized me. I was filled with a horror that I can only call unquenchable. The stench of death never left me.

Each ambush robbed me of sleep, stripped me of pleasures, tormented me with worry, filled me with self-doubt. The loss of my ability to rest was soon followed by the loss of my ability to read. Because I couldn't make the decision to pick up a book, or to open it. I couldn't make any decision at all. Would I like a cup of tea? I had no idea. I barely knew whether to get up in the morning, let alone bother to get dressed. The future? It didn't exist. Everything I thought I had known or cared about suddenly had no meaning. Much of the day I simply concentrated on trying not to blink, since I had noticed the images that hovered over me, waiting to kidnap my mind, were quick to pounce when I closed my eyes.

One hot summer morning my mind was pursued by rotting body fragments. There were intestines. Spongy livers. Hearts that did not beat. Hands. Here was one wearing a wedding ring. I had to prise it off to read the inscription so that I could find out whose hand it was. The clawing stench of decay took my breath away.

I thought it was better to die than live like this.

But how?

Railway lines are quick but they are selfish. People who appear in front of trains cause trauma for the driver and create an unforgettable mess which will torment loved ones for ever. Hanging might not work, or not very quickly. A gun would be good, but how could I get one? Driving my car off a cliff seemed like a clean option. I'd have to find a suitable, accessible cliff, though. Difficult when I barely felt able to change out of second without crashing the gears.

I don't know what I was doing or saying because I could only see the world from inside my head, and it was not a world in which anyone would want to go on living. My actions, whatever they were, greatly alarmed Linda. I was taken, unprotestingly, to A&E, where I was referred to a psychiatric team. Sane, sensible, senior pathologist Dr Richard Shepherd sat and quivered as a psychiatrist gently asked him to share the images he was seeing. I tried to describe them. But no words came out.

It wasn't a difficult diagnosis. I dare say every person reading this book has already diagnosed post-traumatic stress disorder. Apparently, I was alone in not recognizing its symptoms.

My PTSD is not caused by any particular one of the 23,000 bodies on which I have performed post-mortems. And it is not caused by all of them. It is not caused by any particular disaster I have been involved in clearing up. And it is not caused by all of them. It is caused, in its entirety, by a lifetime of bearing first-hand witness to, on behalf of everyone – courts, relatives, public, society – man's inhumanity to man.

The result of this diagnosis?
The summer of 2016 off work.
Two cures: talking and pharmaceutical.
And this book.

I was scheduled to return to post-mortems in the autumn, but I did not see how I could ever work again. I did not see how I could cut arteries into tiny sections again, or lift brains out of skulls again or examine the insides of faces again or stand in the middle of an overflowing mortuary after another disaster with a queue of the dead waiting for me. Again and again and again. My future as a forensic pathologist was unimaginable.

Then, there was a change, small at first. I started to talk. I remembered how Jen and I had sat together in the counselling room in Clapham all those years ago, how my mind had wandered but my mouth had stayed, for the most part, closed. Now, in a quiet room with a sympathetic professional, I allowed my mind to wander – just a little bit at first – and then told the professional where I'd been. It was a dangerous game, letting my mind stroll off where it would. Because God knows what it would get up to if I didn't keep it firmly under control. But with a professional in attendance I, very slowly, week by week, controlled the release of my thoughts. And I found that, by reporting on my excursions to hell, they became fewer. Bit by bit.

One day, quite recently, I began to feel better. There was still no word from the GMC and I really had no idea where the summer had gone or how it had become autumn but suddenly, almost as suddenly as that first panic attack over Hungerford, my acute anxiety lifted. The massive boulder that was going to roll over me any minute lost momentum. The dread that had weighed so much that my feet could not walk and my mind could not think, rose up and floated lightly away like a radioactive cloud.

It was replaced by an intimation, perhaps the ghost, of my former pleasure in life. I knew this couldn't last, that it was just a glimpse of normality, but it was enough for now. I wanted to grab the moment, get in a plane and fly it, to feel the thrill of take-off, to rise above the small, the mundane and the everyday. But of course, after my summer of madness, I had been forced temporarily to surrender my pilot's licence.

I burst in on Linda, who was working at her desk, frowning slightly over a child-abuse case that was soon due in court.

'Let's go for a walk!' I yelled. Too loudly, perhaps. She looked at me strangely but stopped typing at once.

And so we put the old dog and the new puppy in the car and it seemed to me that the autumn sun was burning more intensely than it had all summer. The brilliance of the countryside astonished me, as if I had never been out of town in my life before. When we arrived in a wild place, the leaves were so gold and rustling they looked like lamps on the hillside. The puppy ran round and round in excited circles, barking, and even the old dog scampered a little. The world was lovely, it was dressed magnificently, as though for a party. All summer it had been wearing its finest clothes and all summer I had rudely failed to notice or admire it.

Linda said, 'You look . . .'

'Better?'

She nodded and I saw her face alter without moving, as if, according to some secret rule and very subtly, each cell had just changed position. She didn't even have to smile to look happy now. How hard PTSD is for those who have to watch it.

I tried to absorb the hillside and the leaves and the dogs and Linda and the world's beauty, to guzzle it the way some men guzzle beer, consume all I could before the darkness closed in on me again. Because I knew it must. Cured is not, unfortunately, a word in the PTSD lexicon. But that glimpse of a world without sickness – it must have lasted two, maybe three hours – was enough to make me long for more, to give me the energy to reach for more. The next intimation of normality would last longer. Eventually, one lasted a whole day. Gradually the world of colour and beauty began to reform itself around me, like a jigsaw.

There were (and still are) many regressive moments, of course. If Linda had a drink she made sure she put the ice in it herself. Any communication from my solicitor about the GMC investigation, even just saying there was no news, left me incapable of action for a day, as though she had physically pushed me over. In the office, there were some files I knew I still had to avoid, containing images I could not see. Even this book, which I had been writing on and off for a year or two and finally put to one side, still had chapters I preferred not to revisit for now. But the summer taught me that I wanted to finish it, that I did not want my life's work, forensic pathology, to be a ghostly, ghastly secret from the public. Because talking about the things a civilized society requires civilized people to do makes all of us healthier.

Then, one day, the phone rang and it was my solicitor. She hadn't received the letter yet but she had been told it was on its way. The case against me had been dropped. Suddenly. Without consultation or explanation, as it had begun. It had not even got anywhere near the tribunal.

I can't call this really a champagne moment. I had travelled too long and too painfully for that. But a weight did lift. The world did look clearer, sharper, as if someone had refocused my lens. For a few minutes, I didn't know what to feel. GMC investigation or no, a deep fissure had opened up in my psyche which would always be there.

When I told Linda the good news, the relief and happiness on her face reflected back at me and I began to feel something of her joy and then perhaps a little of my own. So many years of service were not going to end in a welter of unjust accusations. I could carry on. If I wanted to.

It was frightening to return to work. I agreed the date, but as it approached I felt that I really could not do it. The psychologist reminded me that I had been learning to manage bad memories. She was right. I could get them out and review them when I wanted to and then put them back in the drawer when I wanted to. They wouldn't go away. But they could be managed. I would return to work.

As I walked into the mortuary on my first day back there was a moment when I smelled the place, when the door closed behind me, a moment in which I lost momentum.

I stopped still.

I could not go forward. And I could not go back. It was unbearable to enter, unthinkable to run away. I hovered, my mind clouding. And at that moment, the police officers arrived.

'Hello, Doc, good to see you again, how are you?'

I couldn't turn back now. But I didn't have to move on either, we were going to greet each other and talk right here. I stayed put.

The detective was a man I knew and liked. He said, 'Got a very strange case for you today, looking forward to seeing what you make of it.'

A very strange case, eh? It must have been those words that propelled me forward. Five minutes later I was sitting on a sofa with a mug of hot tea in one hand and a biscuit in the other.

The detective looked through his notes.

'Deceased is in her fifties, a complete drunk and a bit of a handful, frankly. Her son-in-law borrowed some money and then left her daughter and never gave back the money, so one day this lady has a few and decides to go to his house and confront him. Lots of shouting and swearing. He says he was steering her gently off the premises but she was so drunk she fell. She said he pushed her. Either way, she ends up on the ground.'

This wasn't sounding strange at all. It happens all the time in my world.

'And did he push her?' I asked.

'We think he did. Although initially his new girlfriend said he didn't – and she's the only witness.'

Nothing strange yet.

I could hear the clangs of the fridge doors as bodies were rolled in and out of them. I swallowed. The sound evoked many disasters, many bodies. I tried to concentrate on the detective.

'The question for you, Doc, is: if he pushed her over, is that what killed her?'

'So how long after the fall did she die?'

'Days and days. She's on the ground and she can't get up. He calls an ambulance. The hospital tells her she's got a fracture in her pelvis and there's not much anyone can do about that. Just keep taking the painkillers. That's the normal treatment. And the fact is, she was shouting and swearing at the staff in A&E and they couldn't get rid of her fast enough . . .'

Was this going to turn into a medical negligence case? I took a sip of tea. It was beginning to get interesting.

'She goes to stay with the daughter, where she's given lots and lots of her favourite tipple. But she's in agony and no amount of booze and painkillers help. Finally, a few days later, the daughter calls an ambulance. Different hospital this time. They say she has not one but five fractures of the pelvis and needs to stay in. But she's gasping for breath and the orthopaedic team decide that she should go to a medical ward because her asthma's so bad.'

'And the medical team agreed? More fool them. So she's an asthmatic alcoholic with a badly broken pelvis?'

'I think she's epileptic as well, actually . . .' The detective passed me the hospital notes and continued while I glanced at the file. Osteoporosis. Asthma. Alcoholism. Epilepsy . . .

'Oh, and diabetes too,' I said.

'This woman was a death waiting to happen,' said one of the police officers. 'She sounds like a medical dictionary.'

The detective was quick: 'But that doesn't mean she died of natural causes.'

'It doesn't,' I agreed. 'So, what happened next?'

'Well, on the medical ward they notice that she has extreme coughing fits and they treat her for asthma and a chest infection. She coughs and coughs, apparently until she faints. After about five days she has another one of these massive coughing fits. Only this time she collapses and dies.'

'What did the hospital do?'

'Resus, of course. They thought it was . . . er . . . pull . . . pull . . .'

I said, 'A pulmonary embolism? Pelvic fractures and she'd been lying in bed for days, it's the obvious diagnosis.'

'That's the one. Anyway, they gave resus and some stuff to, er . . .'

'To dissolve blood clots.'

I was sorry at that. It was certainly the right thing to do but it didn't save the patient and it certainly hadn't helped the pathologist. Because, if there had been a blood clot for me to find, now it would be dissolved.

'We were waiting for her to get better to discuss the GBH charge against the son-in-law and when we rang the hospital to ask if we could question her, the nurse says, "Oh, we forgot to tell you, she's dead." So suddenly it's not GBH, it's manslaughter.'

I finished my tea. Now this had become a strange case. I'd just been presented with five possible causes of death, and it still might be something else entirely. Only her body could tell us why she had died and it was waiting for us now. I stood up. I was curious about this mystery.

'Right. Let's take a look at her.'

On the way into the post-mortem room, I said to the detective, 'This is your department, not mine, but you haven't got a lot of evidence that the son-in-law pushed her. If she was drunk she could have fallen over and injured herself before she even arrived at his house.'

'We've got the girlfriend, actually. She's split up with him. And now she's changed her statement. Says she saw him push the woman over and push her hard.'

Hmmm. No jury is impressed with witnesses changing their statements by 180 degrees.

'And,' he added, 'we have CCTV footage of the deceased about five minutes before she went to the son-in-law's and she had no problems walking then. So what we really need in order to prosecute is your evidence, Doc.'

I would look for that evidence. But with a constant awareness that there was a manslaughter charge and the possibility of a prison sentence hanging over the defendant. I must be absolutely sure I was right before I could give the police my statement.

The woman was fifty-six and looked ninety-six.

'Are you sure we've got her age right?' I asked.

The police officer nodded.

I examined the exterior of her bloated body. It was peppered with abrasions and scars, as the bodies of alcoholics often are. Each would have to be measured and described. I made my notes and kept the photographer busy.

'What quality of image do you set on the camera?' I asked him.

He looked at me, surprised.

'The lowest, Doc.'

I was fascinated. 'Why the lowest – surely you want the best-quality images possible?'

'True,' he said, 'but the police computer system can't cope with big files and so we have to use low quality.'

There was no answer to this acceptance of inaccuracy, and I could hear no apparent distress in his voice. It was from his point of view a simple and sensible conclusion, given the poor computer system. It didn't seem to matter that the photos he took would be used to convict hundreds of people. And had nearly finished off my career. I just sighed. What else could I do?

Then it was time to make my first incision. I stood at the patient's right side, PM40 in hand. It felt like many long years since the last time I had stood by a naked, dead body. Did I really want to do this? Store up more bad memories in that hideous scrapbook inside my head that could still open, without warning, at any time?

I gradually exposed the body, entering the abdominal cavity using a unique cut. Unique because I had invented it. Let's call it the Shepherd cut. Instead of slicing the muscles down the midline, I cut along the bottom of the ribs and down the sides of the abdomen. Then I fold down the muscles of the abdominal wall, like opening the lid of a box. Neat, effective. And I found here, around the fractured pelvis, extensive blood in the muscles and tissues.

'Looking promising!' said the detective happily.

'She was certainly haemorrhaging,' I agreed, baling out the blood and then looking at the body's internal organs lying in the chest and abdominal cavities, 'but none of it looks recent.'

As I stared and lifted and poked, the roadmap of her life lay before me.

'Is that her liver?' asked a police officer, pointing to a small, grey organ lying across the top of her abdomen. Even a layman could tell this had not been a healthy organ for a very long time. 'Looks like a dead parrot.'

'You won't need to pickle it, Doc, she's already pickled it for you,' said another.

The detective was shaking his head. He said, 'Doc, please don't tell me her liver killed her.'

I said, 'I agree it looks awful, but I'll know exactly how bad when I can get it under a microscope ... her lungs don't look too good either. Quite a bit of emphysema here.'

The deceased had spent her life by a very busy main road or she had worked in a dirty factory or she had smoked heavily. Her lungs were dark, quite black in areas, and they were pitted by numerous big holes.

'I don't want to hear her asthma killed her either,' said the detective gloomily. 'And if you say she had a heart problem too, I'll cry.'

'She probably did with this little lot. I'll have to get her heart out to look at it properly.'

'Doc, don't give me natural causes. I'd really like to nick him. This woman may only be fifty-six but she looks really old and frail and he's a big bloke and he shoved her over hard and she broke her pelvis in five places and then she died. He shouldn't get away with it.'

I said, 'Her family might have a case against the first hospital for sending her away with just paracetamol when she had five pelvic fractures. Unless, of course, she fell at her daughter's afterwards and got the other four . . .'

'The daughter's not saying, but we'll get the X-rays from the first hospital checked,' said the detective, making a note. 'I'm not really interested in cases against hospitals, though. She got the fracture in the first place because he pushed her.'

'How could she die of a broken pelvis anyway?' asked another officer.

'An indirect cause of death from a broken pelvis would be a pulmonary embolism: she'd been lying in a hospital bed for days and that means a blood clot could easily have developed in her legs and found its way through the blood vessels into her lungs. Unfortunately, the hospital gave her medication during resuscitation to break up any clots so I'm unlikely to find that – if it was ever there.'

'Oh God,' said the detective. 'We need evidence.'

'Well, another common cause of death after a fracture is a different type of embolism called a fat embolism. We don't know how this happens. Maybe fat from the bone marrow at the fracture site finds its way through damaged blood vessels and into the lungs. Once it's there it can be carried through the lungs and then it can get to the heart, the kidneys, the brain . . . it's often fatal. Odd thing is that it takes about a week from the trauma to death.'

'Ah!' The detective's face was brightening. 'When will you know if she's got that?'

'She's probably got it to some extent, a lot of people do after a fracture, after all sorts of things. It's a question of degree . . . I need to know just how many fat emboli she has, and if that number is significant, before I can say that's the cause of death.'

'When will you know, Doc?'

'About a week, but of course we're waiting for toxicology anyway.'

The detective looked at me. He said, 'I told you it was a strange case.'

I grinned back at him. 'Yes,' I agreed, 'it is.'

I thought about the case a lot. But not the next day. Because I had just got my pilot's licence back and now I went flying. Alone, I was suspended by nothing in the middle of nothing with the amazing feast that is the English countryside spread out below me and, in the distance, the deep, sombre blue of the sea. The plane soared. I soared. My thoughts were as gloriously uncluttered as the sky, as the sea.

A week or so later I met the same detective again at another post-mortem. Another strange case.

A man had come out of the pub and later been found dead in a river. His family were convinced that he'd been knocked out by an assailant and then chucked in the water.

'Well?' said the detective from across the post-mortem table. 'Had any luck yet finding the cause of death for the drunken woman who got pushed over?'

I was running an eye over the man from the river. I had a theory about him.

'I've been agonizing over it. That woman really was a complex case. I did find quite a few fat emboli in her lungs and brain but, according to the research, not quite enough to be one hundred per cent sure they were fatal.'

He groaned.

'I'm going to give as cause of death the fractured pelvis with haemorrhages and fat emboli. For part two – that's the associated findings of course – I'm going to add the cirrhosis, diabetes, etc. as underlying conditions.'

He stared at me.

'So! It was the fractures!'

'What I give is my opinion about the cause of death. Others may disagree and in the end it'll be up to the CPS to decide if they want to prosecute. I think they should. But, knowing the CPS nowadays . . .' I rolled my eyes. 'Of course, finally it's up to a jury to decide if that's beyond reasonable doubt or not.'

'They can't decide if he's not been prosecuted. Thanks, Doc. I tell you, I'll be arresting that son-in-law for manslaughter.'

'The CPS will only let you do that if they're sure they can win the case, and right now they're not sure.'

'What's stopping them?'

'They want me to give more weight to the pelvic fractures.'

He looked at me narrowly.

'Well, can you, Doc?'

I stared back at him over the drowned body.

'I've gone as far as my conscience allows.'

'But –'

'My cause of death says it all. She died from complications of her pelvic fractures but she was already an ill lady with several chronic diseases. You take your victims as you find them, right? If some minion at the CPS can't understand what I've written – and I don't think they can – and they've point-blank declined my request for a meeting so I can explain my findings and reasons, what more can I do?'

'Doc –'

'I've been fair. That's my job, to be fair.'

At this point detectives can get very annoyed with pathologists, so I concentrated on the body in front of me. I had a suspicion that this was going to be one of those cases of death by urination. We know that drunks can be unstable and wobble. Not normally too much of an issue, even when urinating, although it does make for messy bathrooms. However, wobbling can become an issue if drunks stop on the way home to relieve themselves in a river or a lake. Then, if they wobble a bit too far, a treacherous combination suddenly occurs: they are both staggering drunk and immersed in cold water.

I examined the man's body carefully for marks of the punch-up his family were convinced had killed him. A few minor bruises . . . a very few lacerations, which looked as if they had happened in the river. And the crucial findings – flies undone and penis exposed. I was just sure I'd find a full bladder when I examined his pelvis. And there was a lot of froth exuding from his mouth and nose, a classic sign of drowning. So, the man was alive when he entered the water, and then . . . I was concentrating so hard that I had almost forgotten the angry detective.

'Doc . . . ?'

I looked up and blinked at him.

'I really admire you.'

I blinked harder. No police officer had said such a thing to me before. Ever.

'You've done a job all these years that most people don't even want to think about. And you're still fascinated – I can tell by watching you. Here's some idiot who pegged it, probably because he fell over peeing while pissed. That woman was a hopeless alcoholic who was at death's door anyway. And you still care about them. No matter what, you care enough to be fair.'

Behind us the mortuary clanged as wagons moved the dead around. Nearby, in the softly lit, pastel-painted bereavement room, a relative sobbed loudly. Around us the group of police officers waited, watching the knife in my hand. I looked at the body before me. Over-weight, balding, fingers puckered and whitened, some skin slippage, a bit of decomposition, a lot of bad luck. My fellow man.

I tried to respond to the detective's words with a light-hearted, throwaway line. Something about how I still loved solving puzzles after forty years. But I couldn't. Because I knew he was right. I did care. And I still do.

# Acknowledgements

I have been very fortunate to spend my career working in a profession which has fascinated me from the first moment I knew it existed. But it is only when I look back over forty fleeting years that I realize what a crucial part family, friends and colleagues have played. I remember them all but they are, of course, far too numerous to list, so here I thank just a few of them. Dr Rufus Crompton and Professor Bill Robertson – they created a job especially for me to study forensic pathology at St George's Hospital and showed me the path ahead.

The many coroners I have worked for and with, including Paul Knapman, John Burton, David Paul, Alison Thompson, Michael Burgess – they have helped me to give understanding and closure to so many devastated families.

My colleagues at Guy's Hospital, Dr Iain West, Dr Vesna Djurovic and Dr Ian Hill. And, of course, The Forensic Medicine Unit at St George's: Dr Robert Chapman, Dr Margaret Stark and Dr Debbi Rogers, as well as the indefatigable Rhiannon Layne and the ever-cheerful Kathy Paylor.

Not forgetting the staff in mortuaries all over the country for their immense skills so seldom recognized or praised and for their friendship, support and, of course, cups of tea! I have worked in courts of all sorts in the UK and abroad and the court staff have always been polite and helpful. I must mention in particular the staff at the Old Bailey, some of whom I've got to know well during the many hours I have spent waiting to give evidence. And I've always been grateful for their cheery smiles and encouraging words after the occasional mauling by a truculent barrister. The many police officers I have worked with, but particularly Steve Gwilliam: he was a wonderful colleague and we rather grew up together professionally in the early years. And it was he who taught me to fly and opened up a whole new world. The many solicitors, barristers and judges with whom it has been a pleasure to work. And then, of course, my family. First Jen, who was such a support to me as my career developed and whose determination in the years we spent together took her own medical career into areas she had never previously contemplated. I am inordinately proud of our children, Chris and Anna, and of my grandchildren, Austin and Iona. And Linda, my wonderful wife and the constant point in my life, who keeps my feet on the ground and who has taught me to love our garden. Without her love and support it would not have been possible at times to carry on. Plus of course the three 'additions' I am very pleased to say she brought with her – Rachael, Sarah and Lydia. Thank you, to all of my family, for your strenuous efforts to prevent me growing old and even the slightest bit pompous.

It was the patience and support of Mark Lucas and Rowland White and all of his fine team, but especially Ariel Pakier, at Michael Joseph who steered the craft you now hold in your hands to a safe landing and I thank them wholeheartedly for this.

Finally, my current Jack Russells, Archie and Bertie, and their predecessors who have been my ever-present companions, personal trainers and totally tolerant confidants.

# He just wanted a decent book to read ...

Not too much to ask, is it? It was in 1935 when Allen Lane, Managing Director of Bodley Head Publishers, stood on a platform at Exeter railway station looking for something good to read on his journey back to London. His choice was limited to popular magazines and poor-quality paperbacks – the same choice faced every day by the vast majority of readers, few of whom could afford hardbacks. Lane's disappointment and subsequent anger at the range of books generally available led him to found a company – and change the world.

*'We believed in the existence in this country of a vast reading public for intelligent books at a low price, and staked everything on it'*
**Sir Allen Lane, 1902–1970, founder of Penguin Books**

The quality paperback had arrived – and not just in bookshops. Lane was adamant that his Penguins should appear in chain stores and tobacconists, and should cost no more than a packet of cigarettes.

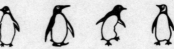

Reading habits (and cigarette prices) have changed since 1935, but Penguin still believes in publishing the best books for everybody to enjoy. We still believe that good design costs no more than bad design, and we still believe that quality books published passionately and responsibly make the world a better place.

So wherever you see the little bird – whether it's on a piece of prize-winning literary fiction or a celebrity autobiography, political tour de force or historical masterpiece, a serial-killer thriller, reference book, world classic or a piece of pure escapism – you can bet that it represents the very best that the genre has to offer.

**Whatever you like to read – trust Penguin.**